Lecturer Practitioners in

Lecturer Practitioners in Action

Judith Lathlean

BSc(Econ), MA, DPhil (Oxon)
Independent Research Consultant in Health Care and
Nursing; Visiting Professor, University of Reading and
University of Surrey

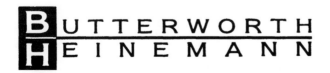

Butterworth-Heinemann
Linacre House, Jordan Hill, Oxford OX2 8DP
A division of Reed Educational and Professional Publishing Ltd

  A member of the Reed Elsevier Group

OXFORD   BOSTON   JOHANNESBURG
MELBOURNE   NEW DELHI   SINGAPORE

First published 1997
© Reed Educational and Professional Ltd 1997

British Library Cataloguing in Publication Data
A catalogue record for this book is available from the British Library

Library of Congress Cataloguing in Publication Data
A catalogue record for this book is available from the Library of Congress

ISBN 0 7506 2449 3

Typeset by Keytec Typesetting Ltd, Bridport, Dorset, UK
Printed and bound in Great Britain by Biddles Ltd, Guildford and King's Lynn

Contents

Preface

Lecturer practitioners in nursing are people who occupy roles where the responsibility for practice, teaching, research and management are vested in a single post. It is clear from the present state of play regarding the existence of lecturer practitioners – often referred to for convenience as LPs – that the numbers of such roles have increased significantly over the past decade. A survey conducted by the NHS Executive (Hollingsworth, 1997) of all NHS hospital and community trusts in England – with a 76 per cent response rate – found that 123 trusts had lecturer practitioner posts, and that these were evenly spread across the eight regions. Some 262 posts were identified in total, where the post-holder had a combined trust and university remit. Whilst the majority of the LPs were employed in acute trusts, LPs are to be found across the community, mental health, learning disability and midwifery.

Thus LPs are becoming an increasingly popular approach to promote effective collaboration between service and education and to develop research-based nursing practice. And as each institution considers whether such posts are the answer to their concerns about the need for better integration of practice and education, and their desires to improve the quality of nursing, questions are being raised about the roles. How should they be organized, what are the advantages, what are the downsides, do the positive aspects outweigh the negatives, what kind of people should be appointed and at what grade, how should they be financed and what training, preparation and support is necessary for the jobs?

These and many other questions are addressed by this book. The focus is a research project about lecturer practitioners which was conducted from the late 1980s until the mid 1990s in one particular setting. The setting included a number of trusts and their related university – where the decision was made to restructure the organization of nursing services, to develop a new undergraduate programme for nurse education and to establish posts which would be integral to both. This was at a time when lecturer practitioners were a new concept and one designed to overcome previous problems such as failed roles – especially those of clinical teachers and joint appointments – and unsuccessful attempts at bringing service and education closer together, with the consequent so-called theory-practice gap. At this time, there was little evidence of such roles on a wider basis, and thus the planners and the first LPs here were considered by many to be pioneers of an innovative movement.

The story that unfolds is an indepth exploration of a scheme that was viewed as an alternative, and preferred, way of tackling both fundamental concerns in nurse education, and in the development of clinical care. Despite the many positive aspects that were considered to accrue it was not without its challenges. These are shared with the reader. The book then sets these experiences and events in the context of developments in other places, and the message is clear. Many of the same issues are occurring more widely – the good as well as the problematic.

In this way it is envisaged that the book will be of value to a wide audience – practitioners who are engaged in similar roles and attempting to achieve common ends; educators with their remit for ensuring the best possible learning environment for students; and managers and policy makers with their responsibility for finding the best ways of providing high quality and cost-effective nursing care.

Posts may come and go, but clearly the idea is one that has received considerable support from a large number of health care and education institutions. There is now a call for more research to establish the clinical and educational cost effectiveness of the lecturer practitioner role. This was beyond the remit of the research study but insight was gained as to the impact that these lecturer practitioners were having in these two domains. Hopefully the original research, and the subsequent work that is drawn upon in the book, will be the stepping-off point for a further consideration of these important changes within nursing practice and education.

Hollingworth, S. (1997) Lecturer Practitioner Roles in England. A Report Prepared for the Chief Nursing Officer/Director of Nursing. NHS Executive.

Chapter 1

Introduction

This is a book about what it is like to be a lecturer practitioner, that is, a role which combines at the very least elements of practice and education, but may also involve management and research. It is set in the world of nursing and midwifery because it draws primarily on a four-year research study of lecturer practitioners working within one institution of higher education and one health authority. However, since the research was undertaken, a review of the role has taken place in this specific location, as well as there being an expansion of the number of lecturer practitioners elsewhere across the country. Therefore the research will be brought up-to-date by this review as well as set within the wider context.

This chapter first outlines how the research came about prior to introducing the chapters of the book.

Changing education and practice

In the mid 1980s, through research I had undertaken on the role and training needs of the ward sister (Lathlean and Farnish, 1984), and the professional development needs of the newly registered nurse (Lathlean, Smith and Bradley, 1986), I became aware of major changes planned by a particular institution responsible for the training and education of nurses (at the time, a single school of nursing but subsequently to become a Polytechnic and then University department) and its linked health authority, later Trusts. A radical initiative was envisaged which sought not only to create and put in place a new undergraduate programme for the education of nurses and midwives – and the consequent establishment of a new role, known as the 'lecturer practitioner' – but also to have a major effect on the way nursing practice was organized and developed within the health authority.

In the course of the post-registration nurse education research projects mentioned above, I had been alerted by qualified nurses at various levels to deficiencies in the traditional system of nurse education, such as the way in which initial nurse education did not seem adequately to prepare nurses for their first staff nurse post. As such, I was intrigued by the notion in this particular institution that new roles – such as that of the lecturer practitioner – might be a solution to long-standing problems. In addition, the institution had a history of innovative work and thinking in the areas of nursing practice and education.

Requests for further information resulted in a joint meeting between myself, the head of the nursing services (the chief nurse), the most senior clinical practice development nurse, and the designate head of the polytechnic department responsible for the education of nurses. This in itself was interesting, because it signified to me the importance placed by them on this as a joint venture between 'service' and 'education'. Each explained to me that these fundamental changes would have a considerable impact, not only on the provision of a more viable and effective system of education for nurses and midwives, but also on the standards of nursing care. The new role of lecturer practitioner was pivotal to their thinking and plans.

I found the discussion exciting, but at the same time elusive. The considerable commitment of these senior personnel to the ideals underpinning the scheme was evident, but the basis of their beliefs was unclear to me at this point, and the ways in which the principles would be realized in practice was uncertain. I wanted to know more about the intentions and the rationale for lecturer practitioners. But especially I wanted to explore precisely how lecturer practitioners would be 'a solution' when, at my then superficial level of understanding, there seemed to be tensions between the ideals and the action proposed. For example, how would theory and practice be integrated in the programme when two types of job were envisaged – those of lecturer and lecturer practitioner? And indeed, how appropriate was it to attempt to bring together theory and practice in one role, when it could be argued that coming to terms with the tensions between theoretical notions on the one hand, and the reality of practice on the other, is an important aspect of effective professional education (McIntyre, 1990)? Additionally, how viable would it be to attempt to combine quite different activities – which traditionally have been the responsibility of two or more people – within the remit of one individual? These and other puzzling questions prompted this research.

Alternative approaches for the study

My initial inclination was to conduct an evaluation of the lecturer practitioner role. However, following the preliminary work undertaken to define the aims of the research, review the literature and analyse the plans for the role, this idea was rejected. I felt that since the establishment of lecturer practitioners was an innovative venture, it needed careful and systematic scrutiny prior to any judgements being made as to its effectiveness.

Indeed, at this point, other alternatives were also considered. I could have attempted an in-depth study of the historical circumstances and processes, the politics, the economics, the social relationships and ideologies which led to the introduction of, and the particular arrangements made for, the lecturer practitioner role. Though these would be fascinating areas for study in their own right, I would have been hampered by the relative paucity of data relating to these aspects. In any case, I was much more interested in examining the developing role of the lecturer practitioner, rather than, for example, conducting a study focusing on the history of ideas about how best to deliver education for a practice discipline such as nursing, or a study justifying the development of the particular role of lecturer practitioner by nurses in one institute of higher education and one health authority.

Nevertheless, given this interest in the nature of the lecturer practitioner role, I still had choices. For example, I could have treated the first lecturer practitioners coming into post as part of an exploratory or 'pilot' study, leading to a much more substantial survey of a large number of lecturer practitioners after a year or so when the role had 'reached a more stable state'. Or I could have studied the role somewhat superficially in this institution and then compared it with similar roles outside the institution and even in other professions such as teaching and medicine. However, none of these possibilities seemed to address in a sufficiently penetrating way the questions that had intrigued me in my very early discussions.

Focus, aims and chosen approach

In weighing up these alternatives, I concluded that my overarching concern was with what the job of lecturer practitioner would involve and how it would be done. Thus I defined my task as being about what 'lecturer practitioning' involved in practice, and established the following two main aims:

- to understand the working lives of lecturer practitioners in one setting as they developed over a period of time;
- to consider the implications for nurse education and practice of the lecturer practitioner concept in action.

In deciding upon the particular approach I would take to achieve these aims, I felt that I needed to understand what was obviously going to be a complex role, rather than take a judgemental stance in terms of my own concerns, or indeed those of others not directly involved. Further, in recognition of this complexity, and the practicalities of the limitations of time and resources for the project, I needed to concentrate, at least for the main part of the research, on a relatively small number of individuals, if I was to understand their role sufficiently. Thus the research was conducted through a longitudinal study of six of the first lecturer practitioners in post (the 'pioneers') over a period of three years, supported by an interview study of the people working most closely with these lecturer practitioners, and a subsequent survey of all lecturer practitioners in the institution. This was set within the context of the plans for lecturer practitioners and the pertinent literature.

Structure of the book

Chapter 2 outlines the way in which the research was conducted, both to provide insight into the *nature* of the study and the findings, and as an example of this particular design, which was primarily qualitative. For those who are perhaps less interested in the process of the research it can be skimmed, yet the rest of the book should still make sense. The third chapter brings together some of the 'theory' and ideas behind the role, and talks about the plans for the implementation of the roles in practice. It is therefore an important precursor to the next four chapters, which present some of the main findings of the research.

Chapter 4 describes the nature of the job and how it developed over time. It presents the reality of being a lecturer practitioner, including how they made sense of their jobs, how they went about what they did, what problems they experienced and what strategies they used to tackle the challenges and overcome the problems.

One of the important aspects of the job was the part that lecturer practitioners play in student learning. Chapter 5 teases out what this meant for lecturer practitioners and the ways in which they involved themselves in the education of students. Lecturer practitioners had varying perceptions about issues to do with theory and practice, and these are graphically illustrated in Chapter 6, including the ways in which they attempted to address them.

A main concern throughout the implementation of these roles – from the planning stage through to the current time – has been the viability of the job. Is it too large, as some people have suggested; is it possible to have a unified role which is different from traditional roles in the past, such as ward sisters, clinical teachers and joint appointments? Chapter 7 explores some of these considerations. The final chapter brings together key issues from all the above chapters and focuses upon the conclusions that can be drawn from the study. It then discusses the extent to which the situation has changed since the time of the research, by considering the findings from a subsequent review of the role. In addition, it sets the lecturer practitioners that were studied within the national scene, where the role is becoming increasingly more popular. For example, how different or similar are lecturer practitioners in this setting from those elsewhere and what is the future for the role?

Many research studies within nursing take an external perspective on a phenomenon at a point in time. It is hoped by presenting this longitudinal study – which attempts to look through the eyes of individuals who are coping with new roles – that valuable insights will be made available to those who are in similar situations, or who are planning to tackle common issues. This is not intended as a definitive text about lecturer practitioners. However, by showing how these particular lecturer practitioners operated, and how this appears to compare with experiences elsewhere, it is anticipated that this will be both of interest and use to anyone with a concern for the implementation of new roles as well as the development of professional practice and education.

Chapter 2

Studying the lecturer practitioners

The empirical work for the study was conducted in one location in three inter-related parts: a study of a small number of lecturer practitioners (referred to as the 'ethnography'); a study of the perspectives of others about selected facets of lecturer practitioners' work; and a survey of all lecturer practitioners. These three parts were supported and supplemented by a literature review and study of the plans for the lecturer practitioner roles in this setting. This chapter focuses on the ethnographic study, since it was by far the most substantial aspect of the research and because its design was unique.

The strategy for the research

In order to gain an understanding of the working lives of the lecturer practitioners – the first aim of the research – it was necessary to decide which kind of methodological approach would be the most appropriate. In this respect a distinction is often made in the literature between 'qualitative' and 'quantitative' methodology. On the one hand, the terms qualitative and quantitative research are used to describe competing philosophical views – or paradigms – about the nature of knowledge in the social world and the ways in which social reality should be studied (i.e. an epistemological position). This was proposed, for example, by Guba and Lincoln (1982). On the other hand, the terms are also used to describe different ways of conducting social investigations (i.e. a technical position). (For a useful discussion of this distinction, see Bryman, 1988.)

Several authors appear to adopt the view that research should be conducted within one or other paradigm. However, when deciding on the approach for this research, such a polarization seemed unhelpful. Certainly, there appears to be a much looser coupling between method and epistemological positions than is sometimes portrayed, and the selection of one position over another is not the best starting point within research. Rather, there are a number of considerations to be taken into account when deciding on a research design. Thus:

first, and perhaps most importantly, [one has] to consider the aims of the research and the questions to be addressed by the project. [And] second, [one has] to think about such issues as the kind of explanation, generalization and understanding that is both desirable and possible. (Lathlean, 1994a, p. 33)

Given the prime aim of the research, this clearly implied a 'qualitative' study, since there was no pre-existing coherent theoretical rationale for the role that could be used as a predetermined framework for a quantitative study, and the analysis of the plans had shown the proposals for lecturer practitioners to be vague. Further, there was a concern not to impose ideas that might be inconsistent with what the lecturer practitioners themselves were trying to do. In addition, there was the practical consideration: initially only a very few lecturer practitioners were in post. Therefore, it was decided that the major focus of the research would be an in-depth 'qualitative' study of a small number of lecturer practitioners – in effect the first or 'pioneer' lecturer practitioners.

There were two further important strategic decisions that informed the choice of research design. First, an understanding of the working lives of the lecturer practitioners could best be gained by investing most energy in an in-depth study and by the development of complex, rich descriptions of six individuals as they lived their lives over a three-year period. But in order to see the extent to which the findings from this study were generalizable across the whole population of lecturer practitioners in the same setting, it was decided to complement it with a subsequent quantitative study. Thus a survey of all lecturer practitioners in post was undertaken, the survey questionnaire being derived on the basis of the ethnography findings.

Second, the in-depth study concentrated on the distinctive perspectives of the lecturer practitioners themselves rather than on a multi-faceted view involving others relating to the lecturer practitioner. The reasons for this were various and included the fact that the role was new and innovative and therefore there was no knowledge of the reality of the job, nor of how it would be developed over time. Further, as previously mentioned, the plans for lecturer practitioners had been found to be general and imprecise in terms of what lecturer practitioners would actually do in practice. Therefore, it would have been inappropriate to try to make sense initially of the role from the perspectives of others, far less evaluate its effectiveness, until there was a substantial understanding of what lecturer practitioners were doing, and how they actually lived their daily working lives. Nevertheless, having gained a thorough understanding from the lecturer practitioners themselves, it was deemed of value to follow the main study with a derivative study to explore the extent to which their understandings were shared by those people working most closely with them.

Having made the decision to have an in-depth intensive study of the first lecturer practitioners as the focus for the research, this led to the development of the main research question – what is the nature and the reality of the job of lecturer practitioner? For example, what do lecturer practitioners do on a day-to-day basis in their jobs? What is the balance between the different aspects of the job? What are the benefits and conversely the challenges of the job? What strategies have been employed in order to cope with or ameliorate the problems and conflicts as well as those to develop the positive aspects?

The ethnographic approach: principles underlying the study

Importantly, the intention of the study was to access the day-to-day experiences, the practices, the logic and the commonsense of lecturer practitioners at work, aspects that form the core of an 'ethnography'. The term 'ethnography' has been conceived in various ways, and the practice of doing an ethnographic study is very broad. Historically, early studies labelled as such were commonly found in anthropology. Essentially, the emphasis was on 'qualitative' understandings of groups and cultures, rather than on the quantification and measurement of known variables.

Hammersley and Atkinson (1983) pointed out that there is disagreement amongst proponents of ethnography about the terminology and about its distinctive feature or features. Some authors, for example, Denzin (1978), use the term 'participant observation' as a cognate term for ethnography, and in preference to it, since it is argued that 'the method involves sharing in people's lives while attempting to learn their symbolic world' (Silverman, 1985). Spradley (1980), in his classic ethnographic studies of tramps, urban nomads and cocktail waitresses, argued that its distinguishing feature is the elicitation of cultural knowledge. Similarly, Aamodt (1991) suggested that ethnography 'attempts to learn what knowledge people use to interpret experience and mould their behaviour within their culturally constituted environment'. Patton (1990), too, presented it as one form or variety of qualitative research which addresses the central question 'what is the culture of this group of people?'. On the other hand, Gumpertz (1981) saw it as the detailed investigation of patterns of social interaction, and Lutz (1981), the holistic analysis of societies. By some writers

> ethnography is portrayed as essentially descriptive, or perhaps a form of story-telling (Walker, 1981); occasionally, by contrast, great emphasis is laid on the development and testing of theory (Glaser and Strauss, 1967) (Denzin, 1978). (Hammersley and Atkinson, 1983, p. 1)

One of the most persuasive descriptions of ethnography, which encapsulates the approach taken in this study, is that of Atkinson and Hammersley. They suggested that in practical terms ethnography is usually taken to refer to social research that has a substantial number of the following features:

> A strong emphasis on exploring the particular phenomena, rather than setting out to test hypotheses about them; a tendency to work primarily with 'unstructured' data, that is, data that have not been coded at the point of data collection in terms of a closed set of analytic categories; investigation of a small number of cases, perhaps just one case in detail; analysis of data that involves explicit interpretation of the meanings and functions of human actions, the product of which mainly takes the form of verbal descriptions, with quantification and statistical analysis playing a subordinate role at most. (Atkinson and Hammersley, 1994, p. 248)

However, in concurring with this description, in this study the ethnography should not be construed as simply equivalent to qualitative method. This kind of distinction may be adequate in some studies, but was not particularly helpful in this research, since it does not highlight with sufficient rigour the underlying principles and practices that were adopted.

Ethnography has often been characterised by a particular theoretical stance, such as an interactionist approach (see, for example, Gumpertz, 1981, in education and Melia, 1982, 1987, in nursing). Silverman (1985) described three approaches to ethnography, each underpinned by a particular theoretical position (namely anthropological, interactionist and ethnomethodological ethnography) but suggests a move towards 'an integrated model of ethnography' which is not specific to any one theoretical model (Silverman, 1985). Such an eclectic and 'non-sectarian version of research practice' (to use Silverman's description) was favoured in this study since the intention was not to adopt one particular theoretical framework. Rather, the strategy employed draws on a number of different versions, and has its own distinctive characteristics. This is in line with many of the 'modern' ethnographies which are based on a set of principles rather than a narrowly defined approach.

Methodologically this study bears some similarity to other research studies in nursing by Benner (1984), MacLeod (1990) and Cahill (1993). These sought to explore the nature of expertise in nursing through the use of 'interpretive' approaches from a hermeneutic phenomenological perspective. Whilst the study of lecturer practitioners is not cast specifically within a phenomenological tradition (e.g. the work of Schutz and Heidegger), it shares both the general aspirations and some of the principles and procedures of work within this tradition, concerned as it is with how people make sense of their lives.

The researcher's role as ethnographer

The way in which the researcher construes his or her role as ethnographer is clearly important. In classic ethnographies, the researcher attempts to go into the fieldwork with 'a conscious attitude of almost complete ignorance' (Spradley, 1979) even though, in reality, they may not be naïve. The notion of the researcher acting as a stranger to the situation is often referred to in the ethnographic literature. For example, Schutz (1964) discussed this at length in his seminal work 'The Stranger', and Agar's (1980) text on ethnography also has the term in its title 'The Professional Stranger'.

There are clearly advantages to this stance in that, in adopting this position, the researcher tries to distance himself from the lives of those that he is seeking to understand, in order not to impose his own conceptions on the situation. In this way, it could be argued, the researcher will be more open to the experiences, behaviours and preoccupations of the participants, rather than being unduly influenced by his own concerns. Nevertheless, there are inevitably limits to this process. Bulmer (1979) doubted whether the researcher is capable of suspending his awareness of relevant theories and concepts, and in any case the researcher brings with them to the research understandings that can be used productively.

In this study, as well as the researcher having prior general knowledge, she knew two of the lecturer practitioners before commencement of the study and had built a relationship with them. It was therefore difficult for them to treat the researcher as a stranger when they already knew her both as a 'friend' and as someone familiar to the world of nursing and nurse education. In addition, during the ethnography, there was a tendency for them to presume the researcher knew from previous experience what was going on, rather than explain things to her as if she were a layperson.

Schutz (1972) argued that it is important to define the limits of suspension of knowledge clearly in terms of the boundaries within which one is working as a social scientist, and the extent to which one either can or should 'act as a stranger' needs careful consideration. This was tackled in three main, linked ways in the ethnography. First, the researcher tried to remain conscious of the desire to acknowledge her prior understanding of the general context of nursing and education, whilst suspending any preconceptions she may have had of the lecturer practitioner role and adopting an attitude of 'ignorance' in relation to it.

Second, it was evident that in some senses the researcher, though external to the particular institutions involved, was an 'insider' to the situation, through her previous knowledge and relationships. Instead of attempting to minimize or overcome this fact, it was used in a positive way, especially in terms of gaining access – both actual and conceptual. To elaborate, it can be easier for the researcher with some 'inside' knowledge of, and acceptance within, a 'culture' both to gain access to participants and to understand what they are talking about. When planning the research and 'recruiting' participants, the partial 'insider' status of the researcher was helpful in that she had some credibility, it facilitated access and made the research processes easier, such as the negotiation with individuals. However, during the ethnography there was the danger of the researcher 'taking things for granted' because of this familiarity, and assuming certain ways of thinking on the part of the lecturer practitioners. Therefore, the researcher had to make constant checks on herself to ensure that she was 'standing back' sufficiently from them in an attempt to understand *their* distinctive ways of thinking. Further, the researcher followed the maxim in grounded theory suggested by Strauss and Corbin (1990) – that of maintaining an attitude of scepticism.

Third, the notion of the researcher as a 'learner' or 'novice' was found to be especially helpful in achieving the necessary 'strangeness'. Some authors have suggested that the researcher plays a particular role whereby she or he seeks to learn from others and to be taught by them. Agar (1980) referred to this as the 'student–child–apprentice learning role of the ethnographer' and Spradley (1979) argued that researchers work together with informants (as opposed to 'subjects', 'respondents' or 'actors'), to produce a cultural description, with the informant being the teacher, and the researcher, the novice. According to Lofland and Lofland (1984), the researcher must put himself into the position of being an 'acceptable incompetent', and thus in need of being informed. However, importantly the difference between the 'lay' novice or incompetent and the researcher is that the latter 'attempts to maintain a self-conscious awareness of what is learned, how it has been learned, and the social transactions that inform the production of such knowledge' (Hammersley and Atkinson, 1983, p. 89). These ideas were consciously employed throughout the study, and proved to be a useful way of getting the respondents to expound and explain their perspectives to the researcher, without taking for granted her knowledge.

Validity and the use of multiple methods

The validity of the study, and particularly the use of multiple methods to ensure this, along with the ability to generalize the findings, were key issues. A distinction is sometimes made between internal validity – the extent to which the research findings represent reality – and external validity – the extent to which abstractions and concepts are applicable across groups. The claim of ethnography to high internal validity derives from the data collection and analysis used (Denzin, 1978). Participant observation over relatively long periods allows for continual data analysis and refinement of constructs, and provides opportunities to ensure the match between categories and participants' reality.

LeCompte and Goetz (1982) suggested that there are certain threats to internal validity of ethnographic studies including: history and maturation (the extent to which phenomena observed at entry are the same as those observed subsequently); observer effects (reactivity between researcher and informants is acknowledged); selection and regression (mainly a problem when sampling of participants occurs); and mortality (loss of participants). In this study attention was paid to all of these aspects. For example, it was important to recognize that in a longitudinal study there is bound to be a historical effect, especially where the context is known to be changing. However, the emphasis in the ethnography was on the *developing* role of the lecturer practitioner and no claim was made as to its stability during the time of the fieldwork. The possible effect of the researcher on the informants has already been considered. In addition, the choice of participant observation as an approach to data collection also acknowledges some interaction between researcher and informants. Mortality, too, was a concern when two of the participants in the first stage resigned and a decision was made to recruit a further individual.

In terms of external validity, LeCompte and Goetz (1982) argued that the factors impinging upon the credibility of the study for cross-group comparisons include: setting effects (constructs may not be transferable because they are a function of the context-under-investigation rather than the context alone); and history effects (cross-group comparisons may be invalid due to unique historical experiences of groups). Just as with the potential threats to internal validity, such external considerations were relevant in this research. Further, one of the aims of the survey was to test the external validity of the ethnography to the boundaries of the lecturer practitioner scheme.

Respondent validation and triangulation of data sources have been put forward as ways of increasing validation. In proposing respondent validation, Hammersley and Atkinson (1983) pointed out that 'some ethnographers have argued that a crucial test for their accounts is whether the actors whose beliefs and behaviour they purport to describe recognize the validity of those accounts'. They further suggested that the value of respondent validation is that the participants may have access to additional knowledge – of the context, of thoughts they had or decisions made – that is not available to the ethnographer. However, they cautioned that it is important to recognize the limitations of respondent validation, especially the false assumption that 'any actor is a privileged commentator on his or her own actions, in the sense that an account of the intentions, motives, or beliefs involved are accompanied by a guarantee of truth' (Hammersley and Atkinson, 1983). They asserted that, as Schutz (1964) and others have noted, 'we can only grasp the meanings of our actions retrospectively [and that] these meanings must be reconstructed on the basis of memory; they are not given in an immediate sense'. They concluded that

> while actors are well-placed informants on their own actions, they are no more than that; and their accounts must be analysed in the same way as any other data, with close consideration being given to possible threats to validity. (Hammersley and Atkinson, 1983, p. 196)

In the ethnography, the accounts derived of the lecturer practitioners were discussed with them in part – but only in part – to test out with them the extent to which they considered the account matched their reality.

A second strategy, proffered by Denzin (1978), is that of triangulation of data sources. Data-source triangulation involves the comparison of data relating to a phenomenon which have been derived, for example, from separate phases of the fieldwork, or from the accounts of various participants, including the researcher. The claim is that if different kinds of data lead to the same conclusion, this increases confidence in the conclusions. In this research, the 'validation' of the accounts of lecturer practitioners' lives was one way in which triangulation was effected. Further, the accounts generated at the three different stages of the ethnography were compared and contrasted for each individual, to examine their consistency. However, care had to be taken to distinguish between differences that occurred as a result of the way the data had been collected and differences that were the result of real differences between the lives of the lecturer practitioners at separate points in time.

In some senses it could be argued that the study of the perspectives of others about the lecturer practitioners was also a form of triangulation, in that it was intended as one way of achieving a fuller and more penetrating understanding of the lecturer practitioners. Nevertheless, caution had to be exercised about the interpretation of results. A match or mismatch between the perceptions of the participants in the study of perspectives and the 'reality' of the lecturer practitioners as observed in the ethnography did not necessarily confirm or call into question the validity of either study. Rather, it could simply mean that there were differences between the lives of lecturer practitioners and others' understandings of those lives.

Participant observation

The researcher in ethnography uses the method of participant observation in order to understand the reality of others. In participant observation, at the extreme case, the researcher is an undercover agent, recruiting him- or herself to a group, and trying to become a member of that group. At the other end of the spectrum, the researcher aims to have no contact at all with those whom she or he is studying.[1] Some have argued that the ideal state is that of complete participation, but this brings certain disadvantages. For example, it can be severely limiting since the participant will be part of the ritual and social practices, the range of data that can be collected will often be restricted, and it may be difficult for the researcher to follow up particular lines of enquiry because of the role expectations. Further,

[1] The term 'participant observation' is used in the literature in three different ways. First, as already mentioned, it is sometimes used as synonymous with 'ethnography'. Second, it is taken to mean the description of the whole fieldwork approach within ethnography and as such includes a range of methods of data collection including observation itself; and third, it refers to a particular type of observation and, in this sense, is contrasted with non-participant observation. In this chapter the second usage of the term is intended.

there is a danger that in becoming a member of the group the participant will 'go native'; this is a concern that is discussed at length in the ethnographic literature. As Hammersley and Atkinson (1983) pointed out, 'not only may the task of analysis be abandoned in favour of the joys of participation, but even where it is retained bias may arise from "over-rapport"'. The more effective the researcher is at becoming a participant, the quicker he or she loses their stance as a stranger, and the ability to continue to suspend commonsense as the life being studied unfolds.

Similarly, the complete observer may be limited in their data collection, what they can observe, and what this will teach them about the individual or group. Thus, commonly, the researcher takes on a role at a point somewhere between the two extremes. Further, many proponents of ethnography argue that, regardless of the overt degree of participation in the setting, ethnographers are always

> outsiders who are partially inside a culture ... Their involvement with their participants is, however, ... governed by an informal tradition that expects a special kind of commitment from the researcher involving sympathising and identifying with the people studied to the extent that the materials produced represent the participants' life in ways that are not just true to life and authentic to outsiders, but that feel legitimate to the participants themselves. (Goetz and LeCompte, 1984, pp. 97–98)

Indeed, in this study a role was adopted which was located between complete participation and complete observation (comparable with Gold's (1958) 'observer as participant' role) in that the researcher had the function of gaining an understanding of the working lives of the lecturer practitioners in part by assisting them to reflect upon, and to articulate, their developing roles.

There are a number of methods available to the participant observer. These include: learning through engaging in an activity (e.g. working in the setting; being a member of the group); observation of various kinds (more or less focused, listening, eavesdropping, shadowing, watching); talk (informal through to carefully set up and planned interviews); and the examination of documentation generated by or in relation to informants. The first is the usual stance for the complete participant observer, though it may be undertaken as one part of the fieldwork when a less complete participant role is adopted. Many ethnographic studies use a combination of the second two or three methods, though some (e.g. Melia, 1981) rely entirely on interviews. Further, the methods used may change over time. In this study a combination of observation, talk and reference to documentation was employed. In addition, the progression was from general

observation, general informal talk and relatively unstructured interviews to more specific observation and more focused interviews.

Selection of cases

Sometimes in ethnography, there is a need to search for an appropriate
setting; in other instances, notably this project, the setting is predetermined. There are still choices to be made, however, in the
selection of cases to be studied, and considerations such as typicality
or learning from extreme or critical cases need to be addressed. The
notion of random sampling, the basis of survey research, is not usually
appropriate, but cases may be chosen by a process of 'theoretical
sampling' (Glaser and Strauss, 1967), that is, they are selected so as
to generate as many categories and properties of categories as possible.

In this ethnography, the initial five cases were 'selected' because
they were the only instances of the phenomenon at the time. However,
they could be thought of as 'critical' cases – using the above
terminology – since they represented the pioneers for the lecturer
practitioner role. When two resigned at the end of the first stage,
sampling was an issue. Thus, apart from the practical consideration of
needing to recruit someone who was willing to take part in such an
extensive study, the criterion of complementarity was employed. In
other words, a further participant was selected who it was believed, by
virtue of being in a different model of the role and a different clinical
specialty, would complement the remaining three.

Sampling within cases is also an important concern. The researcher
should decide what they will observe, where, when and how, as well
as who they will talk to, and what and how they will record. The three
major dimensions of sampling within cases are time, people and
context (Hammersley and Atkinson, 1983). The boundaries of the
cases are also important; for example, in this study, the researcher had
to consider whether she was only interested in the behaviour of
lecturer practitioners whilst they were in a work setting or whether
she should go beyond the hospital and the educational institution to
observe outside.

Research sequence

The progression in ethnographic studies is from a broad frame of
reference to one that is more focused, described by some commentators as progressive focusing. For example, Hammersley and Atkinson

(1983) talked about the 'characteristic "funnel" structure' of ethno-graphic research, whereby progressive focusing takes place throughout its course. This, they suggested, may have two components – first, the development or transformation of the research problem (or research questions) and second, 'a gradual shift from a concern with describing social events and processes to developing and testing explanations'.

They did, however, concede that 'different studies vary considerably in the distance they travel along this road', and that some ethnographies are 'heavily descriptive' with 'the "theory" [remaining] implicit and largely unorganized'.

Clearly, the first stage of an ethnography is the delineation of broad research questions, prior to the making of decisions about the aspects outlined above – sampling, boundaries and methods. In this ethnography, having established the 'social situation' that was to be the focus, and delineated the research questions, decisions were made about the cases to be involved, the parameters, and how the individuals would be studied.

Very early on, it was envisaged that the research would be conducted in a series of stages, though the rationale for these stages, and the relationship between them, had to be worked out as the study proceeded. It was also anticipated that a degree of 'progressive focusing' would be appropriate, but again the way in which this occurred was part of the development of the research over time. Initially, the intended principle for the focusing had been that of taking key themes that had emerged from the first two stages of the ethnography, and attempting a more fine-grained study of them. This procedure is akin to Spradley's (1980) move from grand tour to mini-tour observations or, in grounded theory, the need to collect data until theoretical saturation is achieved. However, in the event, some issues that had been prevalent in the literature review and the plans did not feature strongly in the first two stages of the ethnography, and therefore insights gained from them were used to assist in the focusing of the study.

Data analysis

There are a number of considerations when analysing data in ethnographic studies. These relate to all aspects of the research, and not just to the procedures of analysis themselves. First, there are a number of 'contextual' matters that can both affect the data and how sense is made of them. For example, there is a need to be explicit about the research questions to be addressed, as well as to recognize and analyse conscious and unconscious selectivity in the collection of data, the influence of the researcher in generating the data, and the boundaries for the suspension of preconceptions.

Second, there are requirements in respect of the handling of the data, such as the need to recognize the potential situational specificity of the data collected, and the distinctiveness of each group or individual's preconceptions, common sense, use of language, logic of action and culture. Another consideration is the validation of data and the researcher's interpretation of it by checking across situations, informants and types of data, in addition to validating theorized accounts with the participants themselves.

Third, in terms of the presentation of the analysis, there is the need to justify all concepts and explanations used by reference to the data gathered (in ethnographic accounts, this is usually achieved by the use of verbatim quotes), to deal comprehensively and not selectively with the data collected and not to take 'the obvious' for granted. Further, it is important to provide theorized accounts (referred to as second order accounts) which show the talk and actions of the informants as rational and internally consistent within the frameworks of their own understandings and values. Also it is necessary to give descriptions which are sufficiently explicit for readers to be able to test their relevance and their generalizability to their own situations. These principles informed the procedures adopted for the data analysis in the ethnography.

When seeking procedures for the analysis, it was recognized that, as LeCompte and Goetz (1982) pointed out, 'the analytic processes from which ethnographies are constructed are often vague, intuitive and personalistic'. A number of alternative 'systems' and techniques were considered: for example, Pelto and Pelto's (1978) notion of deductive, inductive and abductive strategies; typological analyses (Lofland, 1971; Lofland and Lofland, 1984); and the 'constant comparative method' of analysis (Glaser and Strauss, 1967). Also, Spradley's (1980) four different – and progressive – types of analysis were examined: domain analysis (a search for larger units of cultural knowledge); taxonomic analysis (a search for the internal structure of the domains, leading to the identification of contrasting sets); componential analysis (a search for attributes that signal differences amongst symbols in a domain); and theme analysis (a search for the relationship among domains and how they are linked to the whole).

This seemed as though it might be appropriate, though it was difficult to see the precise distinctions between the types of analysis and how it might be used in practice in this ethnography. Hammersley and Atkinson's (1983) more generalized approach to analysis in ethnography was also considered. They suggested that the process of analysis begins with the careful reading of, and familiarization with, the data gained. This proceeds to the identification of interesting patterns, surprising notions, and the relationships of the data to common-sense knowledge and previous theory. The analyst then looks at

> whether there are any apparent inconsistencies or contradictions between the views of different groups or individuals, or between people's expressed beliefs or attitudes. (Hammersley and Atkinson, 1983, p. 178)

A method of analysis was developed especially for this project which draws in particular on the ideas of Hammersley and Atkinson (1983), Silverman (1985) and Spradley (1980), as well as bearing some similarity to a grounded theory approach to data analysis. The principles in each of the three stages included the collection of first order data from the lecturer practitioners – both observational and through interviews – and the generation of second order accounts for each person which were deemed to be faithful to the distinctions, connections and emphases of the individuals. These accounts were then validated with individuals. The final stage of analysis entailed the synthesizing of the separate accounts, and the search for common patterns as well as differences. The synthesized accounts from the second and third stages were compared with the previous stage in order to confirm similarities or to ascertain changes.

Conducting the ethnographic study

The ethnographic study of individual lecturer practitioners was conducted in three chronological stages, which are summarized in Figure 1.

Since at the start of the research the job of lecturer practitioner had not been fully established and institutionalised in the setting under study and, at the time of the selection, very few lecturer practitioners had been appointed, neither typicality nor randomness was an appropriate basis for the choice of cases. From preliminary observations, it was apparent that there were only six people occupying full or 'designate' lecturer practitioner roles prior to the start of the fieldwork. One had to be excluded for personal reasons and the other five were approached with a view to taking part in the study. It was evident that these five were not only pioneers, in the sense that they had often negotiated their appointment and written their own job descriptions, but also they were following different models of the role (see Chapter 3). The participants will be referred to as Ann, Beth, Charlotte, David and Ellen – fictitious names to preserve anonymity.

Phase 1
The fieldwork was undertaken from June 1989 to August 1990.
  It comprised the study of five lecturer practitioners in the early part of their jobs. Four were observed and asked questions about the observations, and the fifth was mainly interviewed. The purpose was to gain a very detailed account of the lives of the five.

Phase 2
The fieldwork was undertaken from September 1990 to September 1991.
  Four lecturer practitioners were studied – three original and one newly recruited. All were observed and interviewed about the observations. The purpose was to continue with the detailed account at a more developed stage in the lives of the four, and when all had students on their wards.

Phase 3
The fieldwork was undertaken from September 1991 to March 1992.
  Four lecturer practitioners were studied. All were observed and interviewed about the observations. The purpose was to update the accounts gained in the previous stages, and especially to focus in more depth on certain key elements that either had emerged from them or were important in the plans or literature review.

Figure 1 Summary of the main stages of the ethnographic study

All five individuals were approached directly and asked if they would be willing to take part in the study. The study was described to them as

a study of the working lives of [five] lecturer practitioners, in which I, as the researcher, am trying to learn what it is like to be a lecturer practitioner.

The role of the researcher was raised with them, and the involvement that it was likely to entail for the participants was considered. The confidentiality of the information gained was stressed. All five agreed to participate.

By the end of the first stage, two of the lecturer practitioners – Charlotte and David – had resigned, and obviously could no longer form part of the ongoing study, though both had agreed to comment on the accounts generated about their jobs. A decision had then to be made about whether to continue only with the remaining three lecturer practitioners, or recruit other lecturer practitioners. There were alternatives. Either it could have been argued that the three cases would have been sufficient to provide rich, descriptive accounts of being a lecturer practitioner, and an adequate basis for theorization. However, at this point, the educational aspects of the role of lecturer practitioner had barely been explored and, of the three remaining participants, two were occupying very similar roles. Therefore, mainly on the grounds that an important part of their lives had yet to be understood, and that much is to be gained by the study of contrasting cases (Mitchell, 1983), a further lecturer practitioner was recruited – Felicity. She was selected mainly for two reasons: she was working in a different field – paediatrics, whereas the others had all been in the adult nursing field – and she seemed to be in quite a different model of the role. In addition, she was keen to participate.

The first stage of the ethnographic study

The purpose of the first part of the ethnography was, using Spradley's terminology, to conduct a 'grand tour' of the working lives of the five lecturer practitioners. The grand tour comprised an overview of each of the five, gained without undue probing, in order to map out the totality of their jobs in their terms.

The role of the researcher

The principles underpinning the role of and stance adopted by the researcher in this study have already been outlined. The researcher accepted that in many ways she was an 'insider', and used the positive aspects of this. However, the advantages of being a stranger, or perhaps more accurately acting like a novice, were also appreciated and the researcher took steps to maximize these. For example, she explained to the participants at the outset that they should not assume knowledge on the part of the researcher, and, on the other hand, the researcher took every opportunity to check out with the lecturer practitioners that her understandings of them were not based on prior assumptions made about them.

There was an acceptance that the researcher would inevitably influence the participants within her 'observer as participant role', an effect that if anything would increase, rather than diminish, over time, as she 'fed-back' her understandings to the lecturer practitioners. Indeed, most of the group said that they found it 'very useful' that they were encouraged to 'reflect upon their roles' by someone who was clearly very interested in observing their experiences and learning about their thinking. This, in turn, was helpful to the researcher, who, conscious of the criticisms of some about the 'smash and grab' notions of research (Rapoport and Rapoport, 1976), where the main advantages of the research process are deemed to rest with those doing the research, felt that she was able to give something to participants in return for the considerable amount of time they were giving to her.

However, the disadvantage was that of the danger of the researcher 'going native' by becoming part of the culture, and not being able to distance herself sufficiently from their distinctive reality.

Methods of data collection

A combination of methods was used for data collection. The researcher's initial inclination was to observe all five participants for a period of time, to consider documentation and then to conduct one or more interviews to clarify the observations and documentation. However, the data collection proved to be far more complex than that, for a number of reasons. First, this was a new job for all concerned, they were working it out as they went along and it was changing in nature during the fieldwork. Second, some of their activities were evident from observation (e.g. clinical work) and others were less so (e.g. 'office-based' work), and this balance varied between the five – in other words, there were some major differences in types of activity between the five. And third, some felt more 'confident' that the reality of their jobs would be better accessed by one method as opposed to another. In this third respect, it has to be said that there was an element of what the participant was comfortable with, and what he or she would 'allow' to happen. Particularly, two were slightly nervous that observation would not reveal what they considered their job to be really about. Nevertheless, the over-riding concern of the researcher in choosing which methods to use, and in which order, was to gain the clearest and most detailed picture possible of the working lives of these five individuals.

After preliminary discussions with each of the lecturer practitioners, the most effective initial mode of data collection was agreed. With Ann and Beth (and later Felicity) it was felt most appropriate to observe them in various settings first, and over a period of time, interspersed with informal discussions and interviews. With Charlotte and Ellen, the best approach seemed to be a combination of relatively unstructured interviews first, followed by periods of observation in particular settings and then further interviews and discussions. With David, a series of in-depth interviews with minimal observation was chosen, since this seemed to be the most appropriate way of finding out about the different facets of his life, as well as being what he was happiest with. In addition, all belonged to a support group for lecturer practitioners, and it was agreed that the researcher could attend these meetings as an observer.

The methods used were constantly reviewed in relation to each participant. Thus, for example, if it seemed from an interview that a new 'phase' of the job was being entered, or that some aspect had been 'missed', arrangements were made to do a further period of observation. Or if 'saturation' point appeared to be reached following several observations, with few new insights apparently being generated, an interview was arranged.

During the study, other events relevant to, or attended by, lecturer practitioners took place, ranging from formal activities such as workshops, seminars and meetings to less formal discussions and chance meetings. Also, a certain amount of documentation, particularly as generated by the lecturer practitioners themselves, was available. This included job descriptions, papers written as part of the performance review process and personal work diaries. The rationale for which documents to include was based on the research questions; that is, did they help to inform the researcher about what the lecturer practitioners were actually doing on a day-to-day basis, and how they were developing their roles. As such, this excluded documents generated before the ethnography, first, because they were speculative about what lecturer practitioners would do, rather than what they were doing, and second, because these documents were forming the basis for the separate, but complementary, study of the plans for lecturer practitioners.

The boundaries of the cases

It quickly became clear with some of the participants that they did not cease to act as lecturer practitioners outside of their 'normal' work settings such as the hospital and the educational institution. Not only were they involved in lecturer practitioner activities (as perceived by them) outwith these settings, but they also talked about and rationalized their roles in them.

The rationale for which settings would be included and excluded as legitimate for observing was based on *their* conception of what was a work situation. If, for example, they chose to plan a workshop for other lecturer practitioners, or a seminar on research for undergraduate students, at home, then for the purposes of this activity their home was their work setting. Likewise, if they deliberately met with others (other lecturer practitioners, for example, or managers) over dinner in order to negotiate an aspect of their role, or to clarify their role or inform others, then they might well view this as part of their job. If, however, they met socially with others and discussed aspects of their job in passing, this would not necessarily be seen by them as part of their job, but more as a way of communicating with friends. In order to clarify the boundaries, if agreement was not reached in advance of the event, the issue of whether this constituted a 'work setting' in the minds of the lecturer practitioners was deliberately raised with them subsequently. Nevertheless, the precise boundary proved difficult to establish, especially as the lecturer practitioners' perceptions of it changed over time.

There were clearly practical considerations as well. It was not possible for the researcher to be involved with every setting where an aspect of the job might be revealed. For a start, this would have involved a considerable amount of time and, further, the researcher was not always aware of what and when these occasions were. The situations chosen for observation needed to be based on the perceptions of the participants as to which *they* considered were the most likely to provide an understanding of their working lives.

There was also the consideration of what were appropriate situations for the researcher to be observing from an ethical or 'comfort' point of view. To elaborate, it was found that lecturer practitioners were involved in certain activities with patients or other people – students for example – which were deemed, by the lecturer practitioners, to be confidential or sensitive. In these instances, it was made clear to the lecturer practitioner being observed that they could ask the researcher to withdraw temporarily. Also, in situations where the lecturer practitioner felt uncomfortable with the presence of an outsider, the lecturer practitioner's right to exclude the researcher was assured.

In these situations the researcher needed to make it evident to the informant that she or he could choose, or at least limit the settings in which the researcher observed. However, the study would have been impoverished if the researcher had been excluded from too many situations. Thus every attempt was made to conduct the observations in such a way that exclusion of the researcher was rarely sought, for example, by stressing the confidentiality of the information gained and the non-judgemental nature of the observations made, and by the researcher trying to establish a rapport with, and therefore acceptance by, the informants.

The challenges of the data collection

Though initially some difficulties were experienced in knowing what to observe or to ask questions about, these to a certain extent were resolved by having fairly broad boundaries which, very largely, were determined by the lecturer practitioners themselves (i.e. if they said it was relevant it was); by the researcher reviewing her understandings with them as the fieldwork progressed so that she could be sure she was observing what was important (to them); and by constantly returning to the research questions.

As already mentioned, a 'best mode' of data collection was

tentatively agreed with each participant. It was evident from looking at their working patterns that continuous observation of each case in turn (for example, a week spent on each of the five consecutively) would be inappropriate for a number of reasons. For example, since their roles were in a state of development and the jobs were in no way constant over the period of observation, studying each for a block period of time would fail to reveal the range of activities with which they were involved.

Also, at certain points in time, each was focusing on part of their job. For example, Ann and Beth had concentrated periods when they were working on the wards, followed by periods when their activities were much more varied. Beth's role changed when her ward was closed for two weeks. Ann became supernumerary at a particular point. Ellen had several weeks of planning activities followed by weeks working on the ward. David's priority at one stage was preparing for his Open University examinations, followed by the long-term sickness of his immediate manager. And Charlotte had to spend more time on the ward than anticipated during a time of acute shortage of staff on her ward.

There were advantages and disadvantages attached to observing selectively and intermittently. The benefits included the more fruitful use of time – there was less chance of spending undue time in observing the same kind of activity – and the researcher was less likely to become saturated and over-immersed in the situation, to become a central part of the phenomena she was studying, or 'to go native'. Also time could be built in for standing back and trying to make sense of the observations being made. However, there was a greater danger of missing the observation of a less obvious or unanticipated aspect of the job; one could never be absolutely sure that a comprehensive picture of the working life of the participant had been gained, though methods for counteracting this were employed.

The relationship between different data collection methods

The fieldwork for all but David entailed a combination of observation and talk, including interviews, as well as consideration of documentation. The purpose of the interviews was four-fold: first, and most importantly, to access the way lecturer practitioners talked about the observed behaviour; second, to allow the researcher to clarify her observations; third, to ascertain how representative the observations had been; and fourth, to allow the participants to provide additional insights on aspects of their jobs that had not been observed. Except for the preliminary, exploratory interviews, the questions asked emanated from the observations. The aim was to conduct what

Spradley (1979) termed 'ethnographic interviews', which 'share many features with the friendly conversation'. Interviews were often followed by periods of observation, when further aspects – often identified in the interviews – were explored further.

With David, there were mainly interview data, which were not primarily about direct observations. This potentially meant that the data for David were of a different 'order' from that relating to the other four. Various strategies were adopted in order to minimize the effects of these differences: for example, by taking him through his job in such a way that it was possible to visualize what it was he was doing; by looking with him at his general diary and asking him to describe in detail events and activities; by looking through his reflective diary to see what he was reflecting on; and by asking him to focus upon what he actually did in preference to what he wanted to do. Nevertheless, it was acknowledged that the researcher's understanding had to be based especially on talk about actions, rather than on observation of the actions themselves. This needed to be taken into consideration when preparing the account of his working life.

Comparison across cases

In conducting the fieldwork for the ethnography, two alternative approaches were possible. The five participants could either have been considered as totally separate cases, or insights gained from one could have been used to raise questions with another. The first approach is methodologically more straightforward since it preserves the internal consistency of how each case is tackled. In this, differences found between cases should not have occurred as a result of asking different questions, though inevitably the research questions become more elaborated as the study proceeds. But practically, it was difficult for the researcher not to be influenced by the insights gained from one case when observing in another, and indeed an aim was to be able eventually to compare and contrast the cases. Thus an attempt was made first to develop an understanding of each case in its own right and only then to use this knowledge in a comparative way.

Alternative perspectives

As the participant observation study proceeded, an unanticipated concern arose. When the lecturer practitioners were observed in many different forums where they were relating to each other and to others outside the group with whom they worked, there were some differences in how they talked about their lives. Whilst the disparities appeared in the main to be qualitative – that is, more to do with the way they talked and the emphases they gave – rather than actually conflicting, some thought about how to handle the situation was necessary.

There seemed to be two choices. The study could have been limited to the observation of lecturer practitioners going about their jobs in narrowly defined settings, with a second and quite separate investigation being of lecturer practitioners in interaction with each other. In this case, since the logic of the two aspects would have been different, it would have been inadvisable to attempt simply to combine the data from the two. Alternatively, it could be argued that part of a lecturer practitioner's job entailed talking to others about their role and its viability. In adopting this latter stance, the researcher was able to see the contrasts between the ways the lecturer practitioners behaved and talked, and the positions they adopted in different contexts, as well as how they theorized about and made sense of their day-to-day lives when in communication with their fellow practitioners, and indeed with the researcher. This did, however, raise an issue in terms of the analysis of the data – that of distinguishing where necessary between the observed actions and commentary on those actions, and what can be described as the 'armchair rhetoric' of lecturer practitioners.

The second stage of the ethnographic study

It became evident towards the end of the first stage of the ethnography that although an in-depth understanding was beginning to emerge about the realities of life as a lecturer practitioner, this was in the very early part of their jobs. All had mentioned how 'things would be different when students hit the ward'. Thus a second stage of fieldwork was planned, the purpose of which was to address the same kind of facets as in the first stage, but at a time when the job had progressed, and in particular when the educational aspects were more prominent than hitherto.

Two participants resigned at the end of the first stage, and Felicity was invited to join the study at this point. It was considered desirable to make some attempt to understand her life during the period covered by the first stage. Quite fortuitously, Felicity needed to review her first year in post with a colleague. Thus, she described at length what she had been doing, the challenges she had faced and the ways in which she had dealt with them.

The fieldwork formed a similar pattern to that undertaken in the first stage, with all four being observed and interviewed over a number of months.

The third stage of the ethnographic study

By the end of the second stage, a thorough overall picture of the four lecturer practitioners' working lives up to this point had been gained. Nevertheless, in the autumn of 1991, the third year of the under-graduate programme was about to commence and the students had moved from their common foundation years into their branch studies. The lecturer practitioners studied tended to see this as another phase in their jobs. Therefore, it was felt to be important to extend the fieldwork into this period and to up-date the accounts from the first two stages. In addition, there was another, more fundamental aim for this stage, and one that required a different strategy.

As a result of the literature review and the study of the plans, various potential general ideals pertaining to the development of lecturer practitioners had been identified. As explained previously, they formed a general context for the ethnographic study. During the first and second stages of the ethnography, insight had been gained about these ideals and others in respect of the lecturer practitioner scheme in action. There were three in particular: they were to do with the nature of the job itself (viability, unification and differentiation), the role of the lecturer practitioner in respect of student learning and the part played by lecturer practitioners in relation to issues of theory and practice.

These issues had either been avowedly problematic, for example, there had been constant concerns about the viability of the job, or it had been very unclear from the early stages what was actually happening in practice or how the ideals were being achieved. In the case of concerns about theory and practice, although this aspect had featured prominently in the literature review and somewhat in the analysis of the plans, it had only been talked about to a very limited extent in the ethnography. It was difficult, therefore, to understand how lecturer practitioners were providing a solution to the so-called theory practice problem. Furthermore, in respect of a related facet of the theory practice issue, although there was the notion of embodying teaching and practice in the same person, in reality it did not seem to work like that. Thus, at the end of second stage a number of questions remained in respect of these three themes, and further exploration was deemed necessary of five questions: how viable is the job; is the lecturer practitioner job a unified role; are distinctions made between the different models of lecturer practitioner and between different roles; what is the nature of the lecturer practitioner's role in relation to students' learning; and what part do lecturer practitioners play in relation to the theory–practice problem?

Analysis

For each part of the ethnography, there were two stages of analysis. In the first stage, the first order data from fieldnotes of observations in various settings, transcriptions of interviews and documentation were scrutinized to produce a second order account for each lecturer practitioner. Each account was validated by the individual lecturer practitioner, with the following four questions:

1. As far as you can remember, is there anything in this account which needs to be changed in order for this to be a *fair* account of what I saw and heard? (i.e. is there anything here which indicates that I have misheard, misunderstood or misinterpreted what I saw and heard)?
2. Is there anything you would like to change or make clearer in retrospect in terms of the things you did and said, perhaps because you *now* feel that they were misleading or just insufficiently clear? (i.e. are you *happy* with this account in retrospect)?
3. Are there aspects which are not representative of your professional life as you lived it over that period, either in terms of things that I have or have not put in? (i.e. is this a comprehensive and balanced account of you at that time)?
4. Are there aspects that have changed since the time of observation (e.g. are you doing different things now, have your priorities altered, has the amount of time you spend on the different facets changed, do you have different problems and challenges now, and so on)?

A number of issues arose. It was far from easy to produce the account: how should it be constructed and presented, for example – as a chronological account, a totality with lots of parts, or something else? Second, the data were a combination of observed actions and armchair rhetoric. Trying to get a balance between the logic of the observable behaviour and their idealized talk about their jobs proved hard. All were articulate and some spent a great deal of time theorizing about the job.

The second stage entailed the synthesis of validated accounts for all lecturer practitioners to provide one account. In the task of synthesizing, the essence of the individual cases can potentially be lost. This was important partly because of the effect of the context. It could be argued that individual cases can only be understood in relation to a context. Also, the promotion of different models of lecturer practitioning was a critical ethos within the whole scheme, and one of the aims was to ascertain whether there appeared to be distinctions between how lecturer practitioners occupying different models lived and construed their jobs. Further, the lecturer practitioners themselves felt that the logical consistency of individuals should be presented. Therefore, an attempt was made to preserve the logical consistency of individual cases whilst at the same time abstracting a good theorized account – the task of adequate generalization from the cases. This was done in part by finishing the account with a 'vignette' of each case.

The study of different perspectives and the survey

As mentioned at the beginning of the chapter, the ethnographic study formed the core of the research. However, it was supported by an interview study which explored the views of others on the activities of individual lecturer practitioners. In particular, the aim of the interview study was to explore the extent to which the lecturer practitioners' understandings in respect of the issues that formed the focus of the third stage of the in-depth study were shared by those with whom the lecturer practitioners worked – mentors (eight) and team leaders (three), nurse managers (four), educators (three) and students (seven). (A total of 25 people were interviewed.)

In addition, a postal questionnaire survey of all the lecturer practitioners in post was conducted in the fourth year of the research. Some 55 questionnaires were returned – a response rate of 93%. Also, the three remaining lecturer practitioners from the ethnographic study completed questionnaires.

More detail of how these two studies were done can be found in Lathlean (1995a), but the findings of both the interview study and the survey are incorporated into the following chapters.

Conclusion

The position adopted in this research was explicitly one of eclecticism in relation to methodology. The concerns were those that could be answered through ethnography, and the derivation of 'rich, thick descriptions' of the working lives of individual lecturer practitioners. Thus, the ethnography formed not only the substance of the fieldwork, and the accounts derived, but also the findings provided the pivot for the other parts of the study. Nevertheless, in terms of gaining a broad understanding of the concept of lecturer practitioners across the institution, and seeing how lecturer practitioners were viewed by others, the two contrasting, but complementary approaches of the survey of all lecturer practitioners and the interview study of the perspective of others were considered important. All of these aspects were in turn supported by the review of the literature and an analysis of the plans, which informed the methodology for the ethnography and provided a general framework for the research.

Chapter 3

Background and plans

As described in Chapter 1, one of the main aims of the lecturer practitioner role was that of tackling issues of theory and practice in nursing and midwifery. Many different professions, especially nursing, education and social work, have identified a dichotomy between theory about professional practice and the practice itself. This has been presented as a perennial problem and numerous attempts have been made, hitherto with limited success, to articulate the concerns and to provide solutions to them.

Nursing – and nurse education in particular – has seen a range of responses. In the 1970s and 1980s, attempts were made to tackle concerns about the 'disparity' between theory and practice, but isolated and individualistic approaches tended to be the norm. This chapter starts by providing a brief historical overview of ways in which theory and practice considerations have been tackled by way of setting this innovative role into context. (More detailed accounts can be found in Lathlean, 1994b and 1995a.) It will then proceed with an outline of the plans that led to the establishment of the role.

Traditional conceptions of theory and practice in nurse education

In nurse education, traditionally the term 'theory' has been used as synonymous with 'theoretical instruction', most of which has taken place in the classroom in the 'school of nursing', and 'practice' refers to the clinical placement or the clinical experience, usually gained in training wards. By the 1980s, a 'modular' system of training was common. The underlying assumption of such systems is that both understanding and skills in respect of a particular aspect of nursing care are facilitated by a close match in time between the theoretical presentation in the classroom and the manifestation of the relevant clinical situation on the ward.

It was expected that the teaching in the classroom would be provided mainly by nurse tutors (who were generalists rather than specialists), with some sessions given by doctors and the occasional input by other health care personnel, scientists and social scientists. On the wards, the ward sisters, or designated staff nurses, were expected 'to instruct the trainees in practical nursing, making use of the clinical opportunities as they occur on the ward' (Jacka and Lewin, 1987). In addition some wards had clinical teachers whose responsibility it was to work with students and provide them with practical teaching. Further, some nurse tutors saw it as their role to spend time with students on the ward, supervising and discussing with them their practice. However, according to Jacka and Lewin (1987), this appeared to be an infrequent occurrence rather than the norm. Essentially, the role of nurse trainees in most programmes was that of apprentices who were on the ward to work as well as to learn.

It seems that, in nurse education, theory has in the past largely been regarded as a body of knowledge, primarily related to patient conditions and disorders, and the nursing skills required to care for such patients, and that which is in the main taught in a decontextualized classroom situation. Practice is caring for patients as a member of the workforce, and learning whilst doing so. The assumption is that student nurses will apply what they have learnt in the classroom when looking after patients, but under the supervision of a ward sister or other trained nurse. Much has been written, however, about the fallibility of such a system.

The identification and definition of a problem

The problems of theory and practice in nursing have in the main been construed in five different ways: first, major ideological differences have been found between education and service which have had a deleterious effect on the education of nurse students; second, there has been a disparity between the theory taught in the classroom and practice in the wards and a need for a greater integration of the theory and practice; third, the part played by the ward sister in the clinical education of students has been seen as problematic; fourth, the assumptions about the learning potential of clinical areas have been investigated and challenged; and fifth, there has been concern regarding the limited articulation of the contextual nature of nursing and the nature of nursing expertise.

The education-service conflict

The nature of the relationship between school and service has been the subject of much investigation. The implication of these studies is that there are fundamental differences between service and education settings primarily because of the ideological differences, that teachers fail to prepare students for the reality of practice, and that these factors cause tensions and conflicts for students. Some solutions are offered, aimed at trying to overcome 'the ideological divide'. For example, Gott (1984) concluded that the divisions that have

> traditionally existed between teachers and service nurses will not be reduced until both groups of nurses recognize similar problems and goals and seek to achieve these together. It is, therefore, recommended that there should be joint teaching/service appointments to designated clinical areas. (Gott, 1984, p. 105)

The need for integration

Empirical studies of nursing practice in the 1970s often concluded that there was a disparity between theory and observed practice, and that there was a need for better integration. Attempts at this have included that of Alexander (1980, 1983), who conducted an experiment in Scotland in five colleges of nursing and their associated hospitals, the aim of which was 'the facilitation of integration of theory and practice'. In the experiment, students were paired and randomly allocated to the experimental or the control group. In relation to the nursing of patients with gastro-intestinal problems, the experimental group students received a planned programme of concurrent theory and directly relevant supervised nursing practice, while the control group students received teaching of the same subject matter by entirely college-based methods.

The relative instructional effectiveness of the two methods of instruction was tested and, although no statistically significant differences were found between the test scores within the pairs, Alexander concluded from a post-experiment 'qualitative' study of the opinions of student nurses, trained ward staff and teachers that the objectives of the experiment in regard to various aspects of theory and practice in nursing had received a very positive evaluation. As a result it was recommended that

> nurse teachers should endeavour to teach nursing where nursing is carried out, with students who are temporarily freed from the responsibilities for providing service, and that ward staff and student nurses should be taught how to teach. (Alexander, 1980, p. iii)

Similarly, McCaugherty (1991a, 1991b), using an action research methodology, developed and evaluated an experiential teaching model to promote integration of theory and practice by first-year students. McCaugherty (1991b) argued that there are two fundamental reasons for what students perceive as a gap between theory and practice – 'the characteristics of theory that lead it to being an imperfect representation of nursing practice' and 'characteristics of nursing practice that make it more complex and varied, in comparison to any theoretical descriptions' (McCaugherty, 1991b). He concluded that reflection by the students on their experience, albeit assisted by the nurse teacher, was the link between doing practice and thinking theory.

The ward sister and clinical learning

It appears that in the education of student nurses, ward sisters and ward staff are assumed to have an educative function, but within nursing curricula historically this has largely been taken-for-granted, rather than made explicit. Nevertheless, thoughts about the ideal part they *should* play, and the comparison of this with the reality have been concerns of researchers and theorists for many years. In addition, some attention has been paid to the appropriateness and quality of clinical areas as places in which students learn to nurse.

The consensus of much of the research is that the ward sister in particular should play a major part in the clinical learning of students but that her role has been deficient in this respect. Further, questions have been raised about how this learning should and does occur: for example, in a master–apprenticeship relationship with learners, imparting her knowledge and expertise on the job through her 'embedded' knowledge and expertise, through the 'modelling' of the application of theory, or in some other way? In this, is she expected to import the theoretical understandings of nursing practice in much the same way as a teacher of nursing would do, but whilst immersed in day-to-day clinical care? Or is she automatically, as an 'expert practitioner' (Benner, 1984), weaving theory into her practice as she goes about her job?

Research has also recognized the ward sister as the key person in the creation of a good environment for learning on the ward, but again there are differing views as to how she can achieve this.

Wards as learning areas

A broader concern than that of the role of the ward sister in teaching students, or in developing the 'learning environment', is that of the potential of the clinical areas themselves as places in which to learn about nursing. Research studies, such as those by Jacka and Lewin

(1987) and Reid (1983, 1985), adopted a common approach to ascertaining the effectiveness of clinical areas in the teaching of nursing – that of the development of a ward profile, or a way of 'measuring' or monitoring the presence of certain factors in the clinical situation which are deemed to facilitate student learning. Though they do not address issues of theory and practice explicitly, by concentrating on scrutinizing clinical areas they highlight the opportunities provided by wards for learning and thus aim at improving the quality of the learning experience.

Changing the system

Much of the foregoing in offering 'solutions' to the bridging of the theory–practice gap, or the better integration of theory and practice in some way, often focused on changing a small part of the system rather than the whole. In the wake of such empirical and experiential evidence, it has been argued that the only way to overcome the problems is by radical innovation whereby the entire system is reviewed and developed.

Major changes in the way that education for nurses is organized have been aimed at rectifying 'fundamental problems' in the system, especially those caused by students being members of the workforce as well as learning nursing. Whilst an RCN Commission (RCN, 1985) called for a review of relationships between education and practice, and Project 2000 (UKCC, 1986) suggested a programme that was both theory and practice in its nature, it can be argued that without even greater changes to the organization of nurse education, for example, in terms of the roles of nurse educators and practitioners, such statements do little in themselves to overcome the disparity between theory and practice. Also, Project 2000 proposals did not seem to reconceptualize the relationship between theory and practice; this is still viewed as practice being the application of theory.

The development and implementation of new roles

There have been many attempts to overcome theory–practice problems by the introduction of new roles. The main ones have been those of clinical teacher and joint appointments.

In the late 1950s, the specialized role of clinical instructor – later called the clinical teacher – was introduced to help students integrate theory and practice and to supervise their clinical practice. But many anecdotal descriptions and research on the clinical teacher role showed dissatisfaction. For example, Martin (1989) concluded that the role of the clinical teacher 'is subject to ambiguity, strain and conflict, and that it lacks the necessary status in either the school of nursing or the wards to have significant impact on nurse education'. Robertson (1987) identified a potential source of conflict with the ward sister and insufficient autonomy to act on the wards as key concerns. Further, Wright (1981) found there to be considerable dissatisfaction with the role, both amongst clinical teachers and members of their role set and concluded that 'in general they are accepted by neither the school as fully developed teachers nor the ward as fully responsible nurses'. Such concerns were taken up by the United Kingdom Central Council for Nurses, Midwives and Health Visitors who decreed that there should be a single grade of teacher rather than the two (UKCC, 1986), and it ceased to recognize new qualifications for clinical teachers after September 1987.

Another 'organizational solution' – suggested in the Briggs Report (DHSS, 1972) and in the Royal Commission on the National Health Service (1979, para 13.43) as a method of bridging the gap between education and service – is that of joint appointments. Although the job of clinical teacher appears to have been relatively clearly understood, and, in the past, recognized as a legitimate role within nurse education, that of a joint appointment has been much more elusive. This seems to be confounded by the variability of joint appointee arrangements. None the less, despite anecdotal evidence of some successful arrangements, there remains the issue of the joint appointment role sometimes being both experienced and conceived as two quite separate jobs within the two settings of education and practice. Further, there is concern about the degree of authority operating within the role to enable the joint appointee to take the actions necessary to bring practice and theory closer together.

In this respect, Champion (1989), in proposing a model for the lecturer practitioner role, theorized about the dimensions of expertise and authority inherent in five different roles (lecturer practitioner, ward sister, nurse tutor, clinical teacher and joint appointments) within two domains – education and practice. She concluded that the roles are 'fundamentally different' in respect of these two dimensions and two domains, and it is these differences which characterize the roles. She illustrated the role of joint appointments as operating quite separately in the two domains of education and practice, and as having 'possibly limited authority' in the two. Vaughan (1990) too, in making out a case for lecturer practitioners, suggested that there have been problems in joint appointments of 'shared leadership, lack of continuity, role conflict, role overload and role confusion', which she argued, in an unpublished paper (Vaughan, 1988), are overcome by roles whereby the way in which work is achieved is reconceptualized and restructured.

The nature of nursing expertise

The concern in the past has been to bring together the facets of theoretical input and the practice of nursing – primarily through organizational means. More recently, researchers and commentators have begun to address the complex issues of the nature of nursing knowledge and expertise and how nursing can best be learnt. For example, Schön (1983, 1987) made a distinction between professional knowledge as the application of science and professional knowledge as derived from practice, with the latter having historically been of low status. Schön challenged the appropriateness of this and said that in practice, as in everyday life, our knowing is embedded in our action, and 'reflection-in-action' involves making conscious the tacit 'knowledge' incorporated in the routines of practice, and subjecting that 'knowledge' to critical examination, to make sense of situations of uncertainty and uniqueness.

In nursing, Benner (1984) aimed to 'examine the differences between practical and theoretical knowledge; provide examples of competencies from the study of nursing practice; describe aspects of practical knowledge; and outline strategies for preserving and extending that knowledge' (Benner, 1984, p. 2). She distinguished between the novice nurse, whose practice is dependent on the possession of acontextual 'objective' knowledge in the form of rules, guidelines and maxims, and the increasingly competent nurse, whose practice is the result of an amalgam of knowledge and skills, related to a context and decreasingly overtly explicit in its theory–practice elements. She argued that nurses move through five identifiable stages – from novice to expert – in the process of acquiring expertise.

MacLeod (1990), clearly heavily influenced by the work of Benner, explored the ideas by examining the nature of everyday experience for nurses and how this contributes to the development of nursing expertise. She conducted an 'interpretative study ... informed by hermeneutic phenomenology' of ten surgical ward sisters, identified as 'excellent and experienced'. Her research aimed both to understand the nature of initial learning to nurse and the later development of expertise, and consequently to identify how such understandings can inform the better preparation of nurses. In doing so she challenges the conventional view whereby theoretical knowledge is seen to be separate from practice. As such, MacLeod's theoretical conclusions about the role of knowledge in practice are consistent with Benner (1984), since Benner found that knowledge and competence were revealed as expert nurses described and reflected on significant incidents from their experience.

It is evident from these and other studies that knowledge is no longer being treated as a static entity. It is now recognized that the nature of knowledge in the nursing context is complex and dynamic, and that professional education has been based on misconceptions about the nature of learning and the development of expertise.

It is apparent when considering research which addresses theory practice issues that two distinctions can be made. First, on the one hand there are studies where a relatively taken-for-granted 'top-down' notion of theory and practice is used. Theory is accepted as a given body of knowledge, primarily taught in classrooms and as relatively unproblematic. Practice is often conceived quite simply as the pursuit that nurses engage in in clinical settings. Problems arise, however, because there is deemed to be a difference between what is taught as theory and what actually does happen in practice, the implication often being that it is the practice that needs to shape up to the 'higher status' theory. Solutions are couched in terms of trying to ensure that theory is 'brought closer' to the practice of nursing (often by structural and organizational devices), though rarely is that 'theory' challenged, nor its relationship to practice questioned. In other words, as Rafferty *et al.* (1996) have suggested,

> most solutions to the theory/practice gap have operated on the assumption that a closer 'fit' or correspondence between theory and practice is not only desirable, but can be engineered by manipulating the chronology, context or job specifications of nurse educators.

On the other hand, in the mid-1980s, research studies began to pose questions about the nature of theory; the nature of practice; the seemingly simplistic idea that all that is needed is for a known and accepted body of knowledge to be applied to the work of nurses in clinical settings; the view that professional education (both initial and continuing) is to do with learning a set of rules or principles and applying them to one's practice; and the implications that these aspects have for understanding the nature of expertise in the skilled nurse practitioner. Such work challenges traditional theory-into-practice notions, it portrays practice as far more complex than hitherto, it suggests that people best learn initially how to become practitioners (nurses) by 'theorizing' about their practice (Schön's 'reflection in and on practice'), and it claims to offer a reconceptualization of the notions of theory and practice, of the 'problems' requiring solution, and the ways of doing this. Whilst clearly this research is a step forward in developing an understanding of theory and practice issues, further conceptual clarification is required.

In conclusion, the review of the literature raises doubts about the way in which theory practice problems have been traditionally conceived. This in turn led to solutions which were a feature of the time, but they were only partially successful, and still the problems of a lack of integration between theory and practice remained. The general understanding then was more of a task oriented, reductionist view of nursing, but the new complexity and contextual nature of holistic nursing was just being recognized and appearing in the literature.

The development of ideas about lecturer practitioners was taking place at the time when these latter approaches to the study of nursing and professional education were embryonic and were only just being reported. Traditional concepts of and views about nursing and nurse education were being challenged from a different perspective and from a growing research base with a different methodological orientation. It is interesting, therefore, to see the extent to which the thinking of those responsible for planning the lecturer practitioner role was apparently influenced by these 'new' ideas, or whether they were mainly couched in terms of the traditional conceptions. The plans could be expected to throw light on such an issue.

The plans for lecturer practitioners

The term 'lecturer practitioner' was not used overtly in the setting for the research until late 1985, and thus the following discussion about the plans is largely based on an analysis of documentation (much of which is unpublished) and literature from this time to the point when the first lecturer practitioners came into post, supplemented by a number of key interviews and informal discussions. This is not to imply, though, that the wider, and the historical, context was unimportant. Clearly, the concept of lecturer practitioners did not just suddenly emerge, and they were located in a larger context – one that was supportive of the development of improved standards of nursing as well as improved educational preparation, specifically in relation to the closer integration of the theoretical elements with the realities and complexities of practice.

The establishment of a large number of lecturer practitioner posts across the health authority was the concern not only of the educationalists, but also of the managers and practitioners. The main personnel involved included senior nurse managers such as the Chief

Nurse and the District Clinical Practice Development Nurse in the Health Authority, and senior staff in the (then) School of Nursing and the Polytechnic, especially a Senior Tutor for Clinical Practice Development. It was evident that much of the thinking about lecturer practitioners can be attributed to this Senior Tutor, and many of the papers were written by her. Indeed one senior manager referred to the concept and establishment of the role as 'the brainchild'of this person.

From the analysis of the documentation emerged such philosophies as the desire to integrate theory and practice, the belief that much of the education of student nurses and midwives should take place in clinical areas, and the vesting in one person of the responsibility and accountability for practice, education and management in areas used for teaching students, as well as discussion about the role of the lecturer practitioner in the new education programme and the lecturer practitioner as an alternative to other roles.

Integrating theory and practice

In an early paper which presented proposals for the teaching roles that would be needed for the planned undergraduate programme for nurse and midwifery education (November 1985), there was an expression of 'the considerable concern within the current educational system for nurses about the lack of integration between theory and practice ... with a major contributory factor being the segregation between the roles of practising nurses and nurse teachers' (p. 1). Consequently, three categories for teachers within the programme were suggested: 'specialized lecturers in related topics; lecturers in nursing – responsible for developing theory specific to nursing; and lecturer practitioners – responsible for integrating theory from all disciplines with practice from a clinical base' (p. 1). It was considered that the third role would equate with a polytechnic lecturer but that the individual would be clinically based.

The problem of a theory–practice gap, and the promotion of the lecturer practitioner role to overcome this gap, was again referred to in a discussion paper entitled 'Lecturer practitioner role' (August 1986). The difficulty was felt to arise from two sources: the clinical credibility of nurse teachers was being challenged, and the responsibility of senior clinical nurses for student education was not recognized in time or preparation. Similarly, other documents concerned with the structure of the proposed degree talked about the 'need for a theory and practice programme', for the 'theory in the course [to] be constructed as theory for practice' and for there to be an integration of theory and practice throughout the course. An approximate 50:50 ratio of 'theoretical' and 'clinical' modules was planned for the course, with all the latter being led by lecturer practitioners.

The need for a new type of post 'which is based in practice as part of the ward/departmental team and which also includes responsibility for the education required by students' (p. 2) was duly recognized by the Nursing Policy Group (NPG) for the District in a paper on 'The Lecturer/Practitioner Role' (November 1986). The post was deemed necessary to ensure 'that practical placements are a part of the course and that the educational experience offered on practical placements is clearly defined and managed' (p. 2).

Subsequently, in a paper actually called 'Integrating theory and practice' (September 1987), the NPG 'confirmed its continued commitment to the belief that education should be based on practice and the theory underlying that practice, and that, in relation to students undergoing formal training, much of that education should take place in clinical areas' (p. 1). However, what was meant by 'theory underlying practice' was not clarified in the document. It then went on to suggest the idea of a joint role in that the 'responsibility and accountability for practice, education and management in an area which is being used for teaching students should be vested in one person'. It referred to this person as a 'Senior Nurse Practitioner' in order 'to avoid confusion with present roles'.

The promotion of the lecturer practitioner as a *unified* role was a dominant theme throughout the plans. The health authority had had an inclination toward such roles, but the term 'unified' was little used, except that Vaughan (1989) argued that 'the role follows the lines of unification where the responsibilities for practice, teaching, managing and research are vested in one person'. Nevertheless, it appears that what was meant was not only an amalgamation of these different aspects within one individual's remit, but also the possibility through that individual of bringing together both theory *and* practice.

In summary, lecturer practitioners were proposed as a means of integrating theory and practice in nursing – a solution to a recognized problem. Further, there was the conviction that student education should be 'based on practice and the theory underlying that practice', and that an important role within practice – and one that combined practice and education responsibilities – should be that of the lecturer practitioner. Closely related to this, it was implied that theory and practice would be brought together in practice settings by the very fact that the lecturer practitioners would be responsible for running clinical modules from a clinical base. Vaughan (1987) gave some indication of what this might entail, suggesting that 'vesting the authority for policy-making with the lecturer practitioner would ensure he or she could match teaching and practice', for example, tools advocated in the theoretical programme could be put into practice and the theoretical programme could be adjusted if new methods were found by lecturer practitioners and primary nurses. However, beyond these examples, the mechanisms by which theory and practice would be integrated were unclear.

Lecturer practitioners and a new approach to nurse education

Inextricably linked with these ideas was the argument that lecturer practitioners were critical to the new approach to nurse education planned between the District and the Polytechnic. In an early paper (November 1985), a concern was expressed about the inter-relationship between the roles of nurse teachers and clinical staff in the education of student nurses. It was suggested that ideally there should be much more involvement of nurse teachers within the domain of practitioners.

The argument for the establishment of lecturer practitioner posts, presented in an NPG paper (November 1986), suggested that the current nurse preparation within the institution was inadequate, that it should be transferred to the local Polytechnic, receive the status of a degree, but should also produce a nurse who can put skills into practice. The Chief Nurse concluded that this could be achieved 'by ensuring that practical placements are a part of the course and that the educational experience offered on practical placements is clearly defined and managed. Thus . . . a new type of post [is required] which is based in practice as part of the ward/departmental team and which also includes responsibility for the education required by students' (p. 2). This post he entitled a 'lecturer/practitioner'. Although the balance of numbers of lecturer practitioners in relation to lecturers in nursing for the undergraduate programme was the subject of much debate, no numbers were mentioned at this early point.

Champion (1988), in a conference paper about the nurse as reflective practitioner, suggested that lecturer practitioner roles were being developed in this setting in response to particular needs in professional nurse education.

> Practice exemplars and role models are fundamental [in professional education]. This includes modelling in terms of making explicit the exemplars' knowledge-in-action via reflection and in terms of subsequent theory generation and theory testing. This level of exemplars cannot be guaranteed in the UK and there is little evidence of role modelling. Thus in [this place] we are developing Lecturer Practitioner roles. (p. 4)

As well as referring to lecturer practitioners as role models,

Champion also raised the concept of 'reflection'. George (1987) had previously suggested that the lecturer practitioner had been created in part as a response to the need to create situations whereby 'reflective action' by nurse students could take place, and, in attempting to do so, the lecturer practitioner 'seeks to reshape the practice environment to make it compatible with the nurse educators' aims'.

Lecturer practitioners as an alternative to other roles

In the documentation the lecturer practitioner role was compared and contrasted with that of clinical teacher, the tutor who is engaged in teaching in a clinical setting, and the joint appointment. The first two were felt to have limited control over practice, since the responsibility and authority for the management of practice 'is rightly invested in the clinician' (Vaughan, 1987). Lecturer practitioners were considered to be different from joint appointments because the latter did not 'tackle the issue of dual accountability and the problem of having two bosses'. Nevertheless, in reality it was planned that lecturer practitioners would relate to a service manager for the service/practice element of their role, and an education manager for the 'Poly' aspect, but with no detail as to how potential problems with this arrangement might be prevented.

In addition, joint appointments were deemed not to have worked because, according to Vaughan (1989), they were often 'two jobs in one' with 'no consideration having been given to what parts of the role can be discarded' in order to make the whole manageable. Vaughan argued that it is problematic to 'split off' part of their role, as has happened with clinical teachers, or to simply add responsibilities, as with many joint appointments. Rather, the requisite role should be 'dismantled and restructured'. In the case of lecturer practitioners it was claimed that this had been achieved by paying attention 'not only to the role itself but to the infrasystem and the suprasystem in which the practitioner works'.

Champion (1989) made distinctions between the role of ward sister, joint appointment, clinical teacher and lecturer practitioner in terms of expertise and authority in the practice and educational domains. She plotted these two aspects on a grid, drawing the conclusion that the lecturer practitioner role is the only one that truly encompasses the two domains of education and practice, with post-holders having or developing expertise in both domains, as well as possessing 'the structural authority – the freedom, the right and the expectation, to function and to take responsibility for the way in which they are functioning'.

The plans also referred to lecturer practitioners as replacing the ward sister 'in teaching areas'. For example, an early paper (November 1985) proposed that the lecturer practitioner should take on major functions which are normally attributed to the ward sister, namely: 'authority for the overall co-ordination and policy making of the unit; consultancy for the primary nurses in matters concerning nursing care; responsibility for the teaching of nursing theory within the clinical environment and the co-ordination of appropriate clinical practice for students seconded for a module of learning' (p. 2). In reality, not all lecturer practitioners in post have adopted the ward sister role, nor have ward sisters been universally replaced in teaching areas throughout the health authority.

Areas of responsibility

In the 'Lecturer-practitioner role discussion paper' (August 1986), the role was described as having two aims: to identify and maintain the standards of nursing practice and policies within a defined clinical area; and to prepare and contribute to the educational programme of students in relationship to the theory and practice of nursing within that unit (p. 3).

It was envisaged that lecturer practitioners would undertake the actual clinical care of patients as well as providing advice to others, they would be involved in making policy in clinical areas and in ensuring standards were met. In respect of the educational aspects, they would be engaged in course planning, organizing the 'educational experience' for students, contributing to teaching in the clinical area and possibly elsewhere, plus arranging assessments. However, there was little indication from the documents about the precise nature of the role in relation to student learning; for example, was it envisaged that they would ever actually work with them on a day-to-day basis as a 'mentor'?

The validation and course documentation suggested that they would 'work with students (or other staff) in a way that is supportive and that facilitates reflective learning towards effective practice', and, in describing the role of lecturer practitioners separately from mentors, it was evident that there were separate expectations of the jobs. However, the Chief Nurse did describe one possible function of the lecturer practitioner as 'spending teaching time with students, demonstrating, observing, and allowing students to reflect on practice', so the precise distinctions were quite unclear.

Although mention was made of the lecturer practitioners' function in respect of policy development, skill mix and selection of staff, the management role that was envisaged for lecturer practitioners was uncertain. Similarly, apart from a brief mention about engaging in research for professional development, it was not evident whether research was expected to form a significant part of the work.

Models of lecturer practitioner

Whilst the initial papers implied that there was one lecturer practitioner role only, the first formal expression of different models of senior nurse, which appeared to affect the proposed lecturer practitioner role, came in an NPG paper (September 1987). Four possibilities emerged for the new Senior Nurse Practitioner (SNP):

- Model 1: SNP as expert in practice, education and management, with educational qualifications and responsibility
- Model 2: SNP as expert in practice and management, with responsibility for the educational programme, but with much of the education delegated to a subordinate lecturer practitioner
- Model 3: SNP as expert educator and practitioner, with responsibility for the management, but with much of it delegated to a subordinate post
- Model 4: SNP would enter into a collegiate relationship with one or more SNP(s) (e.g. with management, education or research skills) to provide shared expertise (p. 2).

These were suggested as alternatives for senior nurse roles rather than lecturer practitioners as such, and they were based on the concepts of expertise as well as responsibility. Interestingly, they have often been cited as the rationale for four different models of lecturer practitioner, and it is certainly possible to identify lecturer practitioners who occupy the first and fourth patterns. Nevertheless, it seems that the first written exposition of *LP models* did not emerge until later (Champion, 1989). They were described in a schema that was based much more on the management function of the lecturer practitioner, or the multiple roles they would occupy, rather than on expertise. Thus:

Model 1 = LP, WM and URM

Model 2 = LP and WM

Model 3 = LP and URM

Model 4 = LP only

... where LP is lecturer practitioner, WM is ward manager or sister, and URM is unit resource manager or senior sister.

The two schemas are clearly not synonymous, though Model 1 in both is the same. Thus a lecturer practitioner who is also a senior

sister and a ward sister should have expertise in practice, education
and management, plus educational qualifications and assume educational responsibility. This is often referred to in common parlance as
'the pure model' of lecturer practitioner, and Model 4 in the first
as the collegiate model. Whilst the notion of models was a feature of
the later stages of planning, different bases for these models were
promoted.

Qualifications, expertise and role preparation

Mention was made in the plans about the requisite qualifications for
lecturer practitioner, and the background necessary. Thus it was seen
as 'a highly skilled role requiring expertise in both clinical practice
and education' and one that would necessitate 'as a minimum level
of preparation a diploma in nursing and an approved educational
qualification'. This was to be the baseline and 'ideally the preparation
would be considerably higher' (November 1985). In a later paper
devoted almost entirely to the potential requirements of, and
preparation for, the role, the ideal qualifications were thought to be:
'a degree or higher degree in nursing or a related topic, a certificate
in education, and management experience and a recognized course'
(September 1986). However, this was noted as a long-term aim, since
although it would be desirable eventually for all lecturer practitioners
to have proven ability within the three areas of clinical practice,
teaching and management, with research as an optional extra, some
compromises were accepted as inevitable in the short term.

The Course Document (1989) was more precise about the
acceptable qualifications and experience, and about the level of
expertise achieved. For example, it stated that

> lecturer practitioners will demonstrate that they are expert prac-
> titioners in their specialty . . . and will normally . . . have a
> minimum of 3 years post-registration experience with a minimum
> of 2 years in that specialism. [They would] demonstrate a high
> standard of practice (according to a Slater or other observational
> assessment) and . . . on-going practice development and evaluation
> (according to observational assessment and/or peer report). (p. 82)

Additionally, they were expected to 'demonstrate an academic ability,
an understanding of learning and teaching processes, an ability to
facilitate learning and to participate in curriculum development' as
well as show leadership skills. How each of these was to be judged
was specified in more detail.

Preparation was mainly referred to in terms of the skills and
expertise that the person would bring to the role, though the Chief

Nurse did caution, in interview, that 'at present there is no one who is exactly fit for the LP role'. He suggested therefore that 'the development work is phenomenal and that it is important to consider this area and what is needed'. The validation and course documents talked about the need for 'a planned programme of development of clinical and teaching staff', including actual and potential lecturer practitioners, and they referred to ventures already undertaken including a series of workshops run in 1987 on the problem of integrating theory and practice and the role of the lecturer practitioner. They linked development work into the remit of the Clinical Practice Development Team and as part of the plan 'to develop a professionally relevant post-registration degree programme within the modular system'.

It appears that the plans tended to specify the minimum requirements for the role, whilst acknowledging that compromise in the short term would be inevitable. They provided some parameters for the desirable standards of expertise achieved, and although it was suggested that preparation within the role would also be important, how this would be achieved was not described in detail.

Viability of the role

The viability of the role was a feature of the plans, mainly in terms of whether it was in fact a workable role, but also whether there would be people suitable to fit the brief. In the earliest document it was suggested that in order to fulfil the role adequately the lecturer practitioner should have 'full-time secretarial help to assist in the considerable amount of administrative work which is currently undertaken by the ward sister but does not require nursing skills' (November 1985). It seems that the recommendation was motivated in part by the desire to make the role of the lecturer practitioner manageable, but also to allocate non-nursing duties more appropriately.

This was again mentioned (August 1986) when the issue of the role potentially being too big was addressed. Three solutions were offered. First, the role could be restructured so that 'whilst the breadth of responsibilities remained the same, the area over which [they] were exercised could be reduced' (e.g. two wards instead of three per unit, and a lower teacher/student ratio). Second, a secretary could take on administrative and clerical tasks and third, the 'traditional role of ward sister' as always being on the ward could be eschewed and the role of the primary nurses developed to assume greater responsibility. However, despite these recommendations, the viability of the role was one of the most frequently cited concerns within the written feedback (mainly in the form of individual letters) from the tutors, especially in terms of the size of the job.

Notwithstanding these criticisms, the planners saw them as stemming from a fundamental misunderstanding of the nature of the role – primarily that is was not three jobs in one but a new unified role, and that the role would be operating in a new system with other nurses and educators too having different tasks and responsibilities. It was suggested that for it to work there needed to be organizational and attitudinal change (Vaughan, 1990). Further, the expression of concern was seen as a symptom of the doubts and uncertainties of existing staff about the proposed major changes to nurse education, and the inevitable affects this would have on their jobs.

Conclusion

In conclusion, it appears from the documentation that there was a concept of theory-into-practice. It was envisaged that lecturer practitioners' practice would closely reflect the (explicit) theory underlying that practice, that they would ensure a seamless integration of 'practice theory' and practice, and that they would be there – in clinical settings – to 'teach the theory and practice of nursing' as a vital part of the educational programme. What was unclear from the plans, however, was the nature of this 'practice theory' and how it related to the 'theory' being taught by the lecturers in 'theoretical' modules. Further, there seemed to be a tension between the desire to have one person – the lecturer practitioner – as responsible for promoting the theory and practice of nursing for students, yet at the same time having a programme with two components – theoretical and practice modules – with the former being led by people other than lecturer practitioners, i.e. lecturers.

The plans claimed that the lecturer practitioner role would overcome the problems inherent in other roles which encompass practice and education functions (for example, joint appointments). These include role conflict experienced by those with a 'foot in both camps', role overload, dual accountability and authority. Nevertheless, though suggestions were made, for example, that less conflict would be experienced by one person having a double or triple remit (for practice, education and management) rather than being a half-time educator and a half-time ward sister, and that the possession of 'authority' within a practice setting would ameliorate concerns about lack of control over the standards of practice and the creation of the learning environment, it was difficult to see from the plans alone how it was proposed that these problems would be overcome. For example, role overload could still be a potential difficulty, and lecturer practitioners might still be in danger of suffering from the conflicting expectations and cultures of service and education settings. Further, certain models of the role were not designed to give the lecturer practitioner sole authority within the clinical setting: would this be an issue, and if so how would it be overcome?

The distinction between the roles of lecturer practitioner, lecturer and mentor was hazy. In this respect, the expectations of mentors' roles *vis-à-vis* lecturer practitioners in relation to student learning were little explored. Was it envisaged, for example, that the lecturer practitioner, in taking the overall responsibility for teaching students the practice of nursing, would 'delegate' certain defined tasks or functions to the mentor and, if so, would the demarcation in reality between the two roles be quite clear and obvious? Or would the reality be much more one of sharing the responsibility, with roles that were flexible and changing? Further, what were the crucial differences, if any, in relation to the educational aspects, between the job of the lecturer and that of the lecturer practitioner? Would the lecturer practitioner simply be a half- or part-time lecturer, recognizing the obvious implications that this would have in respect of time available, or would the education roles of lecturer practitioner and lecturer be qualitatively different in terms of achieving student learning?

The plans relate to a particular location, and were influenced by factors within that setting. Though many of the ideas emanate from perceived deficiencies within a whole general approach to nurse education and practice, the actual proposals were intrinsically linked to the desire of one particular health authority and school of nursing to improve both nursing care and the education of nurses, and thus took account of local needs and structures. Nevertheless, whilst it was acknowledged that the scheme in action would in some senses be idiosyncratic, it was envisaged that it would be possible to draw insights from it which would be applicable beyond the setting.

Chapter 4

Being a lecturer practitioner

This chapter focuses on the job of lecturer practitioner – what it was like; what the different aspects of the job were and the satisfactions experienced. It draws particularly on the in-depth study of the six lecturer practitioners over a three-year period, but also includes insights from the study of the perspectives of other people and the survey of all lecturer practitioners in post in this setting. It throws light on many different facets, except that the detailed discussion of the educational component of the role, the part played by lecturer practitioners in relation to theory and practice and the problems surrounding the job are reserved for Chapters 5, 6 and 7 respectively.

Profile of the lecturer practitioners

Six lecturer practitioners were studied in great detail: their profiles are summarized in Figure 2. (The names are fictitious.) These will be referred to as 'the six LPs'. In addition, information was gained about the roles of 55 other lecturer practitioners from the survey ('the survey LPs').

In terms of the job title of the survey LPs, the majority were called lecturer practitioners, usually combined with the name of the specialty relating to their clinical area; for example, 'Lecturer practitioner, district nursing', 'Lecturer practitioner, Accident and Emergency department'. This was in line with the six LPs, since five of them had this formal title – the exception being Charlotte who was called a Senior Nurse. Some lecturer practitioners also had other designations in their title, such as Senior Nurse or Ward Sister, and a minority had a different job title with no mention at all of the lecturer practitioner component; for example, 'Clinical Lecturer'.

With respect to the clinical specialties that each worked within, there was a much greater spread with all lecturer practitioners than with the six LPs, since the latter were all institutionally based, and in general medical, surgical, oncology, care of the elderly and paediatric settings. The total population covered all these areas plus other

Ann

Ann worked on a medical unit, comprising two wards. She was senior sister for the unit and ward sister for one of the two wards, thus being, in the terms of the planners, a 'pure model'. (The other ward also had a sister.) She was the second lecturer practitioner to be appointed in the hospital; she wrote her own job description and negotiated many aspects of the job. She had dual accountability: to the Director of Nursing Services for the service part of her role, and to the Polytechnic Departmental Head for the educational part of her role. (This was common for all but one of the participants.)

Beth

Beth was the first lecturer practitioner to be appointed in the hospital where Ann worked also. She was the senior sister of a surgical unit comprising two wards, and the ward sister for one of those wards. (The other ward also had a sister.) Like Ann, she operated within the pure model. She had the same dual accountability.

Charlotte

Charlotte was the first senior sister/lecturer practitioner to be appointed in her hospital, and was a senior sister in a unit for the care of the elderly, comprising two wards. She had a particular responsibility for one of the wards, though she did not use the term 'ward sister' to describe this. Another sister was responsible for the other ward. Charlotte was formally accountable *only* to the Director of Nursing Services. She resigned in September 1990.

David

David was a lecturer practitioner in a small community hospital for the elderly, located within a larger hospital. He came to the post as a tutor from the school of nursing and still had responsibilities for pre-registration students. He worked in an area which did not have a sister, but did have a senior nurse. At one point during the study, the senior nurse left and there was a period of some months when a replacement was awaited. During this time, David undertook the role of the senior nurse as well as his own. Subsequently a new senior nurse was appointed. David, too, had the same dual accountability. He resigned in September 1990.

Ellen

Ellen was within a collegiate role. That is, although she had no direct managerial authority in terms of her designation – she was neither a senior nurse nor a sister – she shared certain managerial functions with the senior nurse for the unit, which specialized in oncology care. At one point during the study, the senior nurse left and there was a period of some months when a replacement was awaited. During this time, Ellen undertook the role of the senior nurse as well as her own. Subsequently a new senior nurse was appointed. Ellen, too, had the same dual accountability.

Felicity

Felicity was the lecturer practitioner for a paediatric ward within a paediatric unit. The ward also had a ward sister. Felicity had a collegiate role, though the nature of the collegiality was uncertain at the outset. In this respect there were two other key people in the unit – a manager practitioner related to a second paediatric ward, and another lecturer practitioner related to a third paediatric ward. Felicity, too, had the same dual accountability.

Figure 2 The lecturer practitioners in the in-depth study

specialties such as ophthalmology, palliative care and orthopaedics; departments such as Accident and Emergency; community nursing (e.g. district nursing, health visiting, school health, practice nursing; community hospitals); midwifery; mental health and learning disabilities.

The six LPs were all contractually full-time lecturer practitioners, compared with 76% of survey LPs. There was no one pattern for the 24% who were part-time lecturer practitioners combined with other roles: the others roles were various and included 'course teacher', 'Macmillan lecturer', 'clinical lecturer', 'clinical specialist', 'ward sister', 'clinical service manager' and 'senior staff nurse'.

Whereas Charlotte and David's roles were ambivalent in terms of the amount of time that each was contracted to spend in service and education, Ann, Beth, Ellen and Felicity were quite explicitly expected to provide 50% of their time to service and 50% to education. This was the same as the majority of lecturer practitioners in the survey, whereby almost three-quarters (69%) were contracted to spend 50% on each. The others had a variety of arrangements including 60/40 (5%), 70/30 (5%), 40/60 (4%), where the first figure represents the service contribution. The remaining 17% provided a range of other variants.

In terms of the grade for the post, all of the six LPs were at clinical grade 'I', or the equivalent on the education scale (grade 2), the norm for a senior nurse or senior tutor job. This compared with just under half of all lecturer practitioners (44%) who were on grade 'I', a fifth (20%) on 'Education 2', a quarter (25%) on grade 'H', with 7% on grade 'G', 2% on 'Education 1' and 2% not known.

The main areas of responsibility for the six LPs, as specified in the job description, were found to be management, practice, education and research. In the survey, whilst 100% of respondents had education, and all but one person (98%) had practice as part of their formal role, just over a quarter (27%) did not have research in their job descriptions and a third (33%) had no specific mention of management. In terms of their stated education responsibilities, Ann, Beth, Ellen and Felicity were mainly involved with the undergraduate programme, in line with 65% of survey lecturer practitioners, whereas 20% of the respondents were primarily involved with post-registration courses, 11% equally with both programmes and 4% had other arrangements.

Finally, with respect to the model of lecturer practitioner that their role most nearly equated to, Ellen was a lecturer practitioner in a collegiate relationship with a senior nurse (compared with 33% of survey lecturer practitioners). Ann and Beth were 'unit manager, ward sister and lecturer practitioner' (compared with 15% of survey lecturer practitioners). Felicity's model did not fit with any of the 'standard' ones, in that she was a Service Delivery Unit Manager and lecturer practitioner. This compared with 13% of survey lecturer practitioners who felt that their model was different from those listed. In addition, 15% were ward sisters and lecturer practitioners; 13% were lecturer practitioners (i.e. with no managerial role); 11% were unit managers and lecturer practitioners; and 7% were in a collegiate relationship with a ward sister. Thus, it seems that apart from the third of all lecturer practitioners who were in a collegiate relationship with a senior nurse, no other model dominated.

The following discussion will centre around the six LPs – what they did in the early stage of their job and how their roles changed over the three years of the study. This will be followed by a consideration of the roles of all the LPs in the survey, and then the views of others working with these LPs will be outlined.

The job of lecturer practitioner in the first stage

The job of lecturer practitioner was clearly multi-faceted and complex. In the first stage, three of them talked about many different 'parts', 'functions' or 'aspects' of their jobs, though two stressed that in reality these were not always clearly distinct and they overlapped. For example, Beth described the pattern of her life as 'not being fixed', with the parts of the job being 'mixed and matched at any one time', and Ellen said that whilst the distinctions, which she based on her job description, were helpful as a means of clarifying what she did and what she was accountable for, in practice her life was not a set of separate activities. Indeed, Ann, Beth and Ellen stressed the 'unified' nature of the role with the inability often to distinguish in reality between the four key areas as outlined in the plans – practice, management, education and research.

The distinction for David was sharper in that he initially described his job as in two major halves – unit work and 'Poly' work – according to the different institutions paying his salary, whereas Charlotte, who was funded solely by the health authority, saw herself primarily as a senior sister, with 'all the clinical aspects of the lecturer's role, but not the Polytechnic teaching aspects'.

As well as thinking in terms of facets of the job, all talked to some extent about phases in the job. For four of them, the first year was a phase in the job during which, according to Ann, 'it has been incredibly important [to] develop a team of nurses and have nursing practice that ... can be exposed'. Similarly, for Beth, this was the time when 'working with staff nurses was [her] priority', in order to achieve the same kind of ends, whereas Charlotte described it more in terms of changing the way that the nursing was organized in her unit, that is, moving from 'traditional ways of working', through team nursing to primary nursing, as well as developing the staff. David referred to the prime focus as being 'the development of nursing'. All contrasted this period with the future, when an increasing focus would be the Polytechnic students in practice modules.

For Ellen, this period comprised not one but several phases. She clearly described these as lasting anything from a week to several months, when she concentrated or 'focused' on one or a small number of activities. Thinking about what she had done, and planning what she was going to do and the time span for this, was an important way in which Ellen 'categorized [her] work'. Thus, many of these phases were planned and deliberate, though not all her plans came to fruition.

All five talked in terms of the ability and necessity to develop the job as they went along. Two referred to writing their own job descriptions and three emphasized the autonomy of the job, deciding upon what they would and would not do, and then 'negotiating with' or 'telling others' such as the director of nursing service, the senior nurse or the head of the polytechnic department. David referred to his experience of 'working out the job as [he went] along', with the problem of others, such as senior nurses, not always agreeing, or having unclear or conflicting expectations. Charlotte similarly talked about the need to 'work it out over time', but referred to her own expectations of aspects of the job not always being matched by those of some other lecturer practitioners.

Two of the five experienced changes to their jobs as the result of the temporary absence of a senior nurse in their units. Thus David was required to 'act up' in a management capacity for about six months, following the sickness and resignation of his senior nurse. And whilst this necessitated the 'suspension of the lecturer practitioner role in favour of management' during this time, it was meant to facilitate the former, since there was a possibility that the unit might in the future be led by a lecturer practitioner. Similarly, Ellen's senior nurse, with whom she had developed a collegiate role, left and Ellen 'acted across' for about three months until a new senior nurse was appointed.

The commonalities and variations in the jobs

The plans envisaged a 'practice' component for all lecturer practitioners, in that they were to have responsibility and authority for both practice and education in a defined clinical area. However, there were only two common elements between all five in this respect. First, they all accepted that their jobs would entail, at the very least, a practice/ clinical and an education aspect, that is, they supported the philosophy underpinning the role, and second, all spent some time on the ward – they were physically present. They described the practice component in similar terms. Thus Ann, Beth and Charlotte talked about working on the ward or working clinically, David referred to it as 'working on the unit' and Ellen as 'being on the ward' or 'having a clinical function'. Nevertheless, how they saw this part of their job, what they actually did in terms of the role they occupied, the range of activities involved in and the amount of time spent on them varied.

All five considered staff development as being an important aspect of what the job was about, especially at this early stage – prior to students being on the wards. For all, the development of staff was embedded in, or closely related to working or being on the ward. It had the tripartite rationale of 'helping the staff as individuals to grow and to learn more about nursing practice', developing the nursing within the ward/unit, and enhancing the clinical environment as a good place in which students would learn.

All five considered themselves as managers, or were involved in the activity of management or managing, albeit that two of them only took on this role fully and solely in the absence of their senior nurse colleague. Further, they all described administration as part of their job, though what this entailed and whether it was a separate entity or enmeshed with everything else, was related to their particular role.

The other facet of the work that was common to all was that described variously as Polytechnic work/teaching, tutor work or the educational aspect of the role. However, within this, the only single activity to be undertaken by all five was the planning of modules in the undergraduate programme.

There were very few major aspects of the jobs that were not apparent for all five to some degree. The differences in the main related to the particular model that each adhered to. So, for example, three of them – Ann, Beth and Charlotte – as senior sisters, were occasionally 'on for the hospital', which meant taking responsibility for major nursing issues arising across the whole hospital. This was not so for the other two. Similarly, the same three were budget holders, whereas Ellen, owing to her collegiate role with the senior nurse, shared this role and David (except when acting up as manager) had minimal involvement. Conversely, though David and Ellen were not designated senior sisters, they were viewed as senior nurses and took part in the senior nurse meetings, just as did the others by virtue of their title.

Some differences occurred which were not related to the model occupied. For three of them (Ann, Beth and Ellen), talking nationally

– or at least outside the health authority – about their jobs was an important and 'reasonably regular occurrence', whereas for the other two, it was not observed nor mentioned as a major part of the job. And three of them (Beth, Ellen and David) were undertaking a first or higher degree and had an average of one day a week study leave in order to do this.

Working on the ward

There were considerable similarities between two of them – Ann and Beth – in terms of the role they occupied when working on the ward, the proportion of their time spent in this way, and the regularity of their presence. Both worked shifts, being 'in the numbers' and allocated to the team that most needed them, for on average two or three shifts a week. Ann tried 'to plan [her] practice so that [she] could do five days in a row' in order to overcome the 'big frustration experienced as a lecturer practitioner of dipping in for odd days'. Even when not 'in the numbers', everyday she had some clinical input which could entail 'walking on the ward to see how patients were' or responding to ward staff on the telephone. They both acted as primary nurses – that is, the nurse responsible for the total care of the patient – in Beth's case 'from time to time', and with Ann 'when she could give some continuity of care'. In the main, though, they were associate nurses, working to the plan of the primary nurse, or even just 'slotting in' and helping out as necessary.

Charlotte's working pattern on the ward was similar to this. She tried to work 'straight days' (from 9 to 5), but because of chronic staff shortages she often had to come in early or stay late. She was on the ward most days, albeit not for a whole day. She too was 'in the numbers', mainly as an associate nurse or providing support for other nursing staff as needed. Charlotte had originally planned to work as a primary nurse on the ward, but this would only have been possible if she could work clinically for three consecutive days, uninterrupted by other aspects of her job. The reality was not so.

David was 'expected' to be on the unit two-and-a-half days a week, thus being regularly in the clinical area, as were Ann, Beth and Charlotte, but he did straight days (usually 8 to 4), and although he had 'worked clinically a great deal', initially because of staff shortages, he saw his role much more as that of a practitioner, being on the unit to develop the nursing, rather than 'doing actual clinical work'. There was 'no question' of him having a regular caseload or acting as an associate nurse.

For Ellen, being on the ward was only part of her clinical function.

Her presence was very variable and, unlike the other four, there was no pattern to her involvement. So, for example, on some days and during certain phases of her job, she spent little or no time on the ward. At other times, she spent whole days or part of a day on the ward on a more regular basis, or she 'did a clinical week' during which she was working as a member of a team, or as a support and a teacher to other nurses, or even, though rarely, 'as a pair of hands'.

Ann and Beth had clear and comparable rationales for clinical work as being an important part of their job. Critically, Ann saw 'caring for patients' as the 'keystone' or 'crux of everything [she] was talking about or trying to do. It was the evidence that [she] could nurse, it was [her] whole reason for being a lecturer practitioner', since, as she put it 'the nurse/patient relationship is the centre of the whole of nursing . . . and . . . if you don't experience things it's more difficult to understand them'. She also used the opportunity to 'monitor what was going on in the wards and try to help [her staff], usually by being there, her presence, and by physically . . . actually doing some of the jobs'.

Further, Ann valued the 'professional and personal benefits' it brought. As she said:

> Every time I am looking after a patient I'm adding experience to my bank of nursing knowledge and more things to fall back on . . . it's essential, it's like recharging your batteries in a way. . . . It's probably the most personally rewarding aspect of the job and the way in which I generate nursing knowledge.

Similarly, Beth highlighted the 'centrality of good clinical care' for the lecturer practitioner role and saw the 'great strength of the role as . . . pivotal on the nature of the nursing care'. For her, this meant that being a lecturer practitioner had to be 'practice centred' and she used this focus of her job to develop the quality of care on the ward. As she said, 'I see part of my job to highlight [poor quality care] with the team, to facilitate some . . . improvement, and to evaluate and feed that back'. Also, Beth was paving the way for the future when the undergraduate students would be on the ward. She wanted them to look at 'excellent nursing' and so she felt that they needed to come to 'an area that had well developed notions of what nursing is', and which enabled them to practise good quality care. Her clinical work on the ward was in part attempting to develop the nursing on the ward for this purpose.

Charlotte was attracted to the job because it gave her the opportunity to be ward-based and to have a regular involvement in clinical work. She saw the job very much as a clinically based senior nurse with an increasing involvement over time with students on the ward rather than in the Polytechnic. Her prime focus on the ward was that of developing the nursing through encouraging first team nursing and then primary nursing.

David, too, talked about the development of nursing as a main rationale for working on the unit. In this he compared himself with a clinical practice development nurse, in that he tried 'to behave a bit like one ... watching, keeping an eye on what the staff were doing, giving them ideas as to what they could do'. He related this both to the 'development of the unit as a good learning environment for "Poly" students', and also as responding to 'the much more human need for the people working there to be given the freedom to develop'.

Ellen's rationale varied according to the different phases and the different activities she was engaged in. Early on she felt it was important to 'get clinical input ... to update clinical skills', to be working in the team 'so as to have the opportunity to work with a staff nurse and plan a development programme with her', to be 'seen to be available and able to give support to the nurses', and to have the opportunity to 'keep an eye on the ward, to see which patients are coming in and to see what the workload's like'.

In terms of what the lecturer practitioners actually did when either working on the ward or fulfilling the clinical aspect of their role, there were considerable similarities between three of them – Ann, Beth and Charlotte. Typically, when working clinically, Ann, Beth (and Charlotte when needed) came on duty at the beginning of the shift and were either involved in a handover meeting and/or in a nurse-to-nurse handover at the patients' bedside, sometimes described as a 'patient round'. Charlotte also took part in a co-ordination meeting, held each day at 9 am, where the occupational therapist, physiotherapist, nurses, auxiliaries and ward clerk planned the day to ensure that activities related to the patient were dovetailed and paced.

The pattern of the day varied according to whether they had their own patients or were providing support to other nurses, and helping out where necessary. If they had their own patients, the shift involved a large number of activities, many of which were related to providing care for those patients, for example, talking with a patient about their condition, the control of their pain, their drugs or the plans for their discharge; washing or assisting a patient to wash; checking and changing dressings; taking temperatures and blood pressures; giving drugs; setting up and monitoring drips; and talking with relatives.

During the day they related – in person or by phone – to a number of other people, especially the ward nurses but also doctors, social workers, physiotherapists, pharmacists, specialist nurses, managers and clinical practice development nurses. The interactions were usually brief, and though they were often in relation to their own patients, sometimes they were to do with ward or unit matters. However, since all three worked on wards with primary nursing, they did not see themselves as 'being in charge'. One of them (Charlotte) explained that in her case: 'when you have a system of primary nursing with nurses taking responsibility for their own patients, as well as some of them having a particular responsibility for ward issues such as doing the off-duty, then the term "ward sister" doesn't really fit the role'. And similarly, though as a more general point, Beth said:

> I don't like the words 'in charge' because there's an element of power and I don't think that anyone has the power any more. It's not vested in one person, it's been divided up to the particular team nurses. Nonetheless, there is an organizational responsibility in terms of bed management and that was invested in the co-ordinator ... though I am not usually that person.

They all spent time talking with the ward nurses during the shift. This could be about their own patients, or because the nurses were asking them about the patients they were nursing. Often, though, it was in moments away from the bedside, at the nurses' station or in the office during breaks, when the lecturer practitioners were, for example, talking with ward staff more generally about patient care, staffing, what would happen during a temporary ward closure, or about current or forthcoming events. Thus Charlotte spent some time talking with her senior primary nurse about the shared aspects of management of the ward such as the off-duty, staffing and the best mix of staff. Importantly, all three used such times to talk with nurses about their own needs – for days off, study time, the opportunity to attend study days or courses, and so on – and they stressed the importance of providing support to the nurses.

The pace of the day was fast, and the three moved quickly from one activity to another, often punctuated by 'interruptions' such as phone calls, people coming to the ward, and queries to deal with. One of the problems of such a day was the amount of work to be done, and, because of this, their ability to give the quality of care needed in the time available. Ann felt particularly frustrated at times by what she described as 'probably nursing at its worst because it's so busy'. She sometimes felt that she should be supervising others rather than 'doing staff nurse work'. However, she later qualified this by saying that she increasingly appreciated the value of staff nurse work, and further that she needed to demonstrate to others 'that [she] could actually cope with a day like that'. In this respect, she considered that 'it lends to [her] credibility when staff see [she] can cope'.

The pattern of a day on the unit for David was somewhat different. He described it as having 'lots of fragments of things' to do, and having 'to juggle them around'. Although initially he had spent a great deal of time working clinically in order to 'provide labour' and 'fill in the staff shortage' – and he had done this in part because he accepted that 'working as a clinician was a good way to find out the ward's strengths and problems' – he felt that his clinical role should be 'to monitor and work with nursing staff, to help them to understand what they were doing, for example by looking with them at care plans, and only very occasionally to be an associate nurse'.

Typically, he would come on about 8 am and listen to the handover meeting at the desk, as a way of getting to meet the night staff and 'in order to find out if the staff (day and night) were all right'. He might then work on the ward clinically, but if not, a discussion with the staff could ensue, often to do with the care of patients and problems being encountered by the staff. This discussion enabled them to 'get to know [his] way of thinking' and him to learn more about the ward. He also tried to meet the primary nurses at coffee time, in order to discuss such aspects as the patient dependency system he was working on, or his role, or problems experienced with the auxiliary role.

Though the senior nurse was absent for a large proportion of the time, when she was there, David spent some time each day discussing with her management issues and problems. He also worked on a number of activities, aimed at 'developing clinical practice on the unit' – a 'very big part of the job' – such as working out a way of measuring dependency, and trying to develop the way the nursing was organized. For several months David had to 'act up' for the senior nurse and 'run the unit' which tended to 'displace the development of clinical practice'.

There was no particular pattern when Ellen was involved with the clinical aspect of her role. Sometimes she worked as a member of a team or even as the team leader or ward co-ordinator. When doing this, her activities were similar to those of Ann, Beth and Charlotte. She stressed that often she was on the ward 'to work alongside the nurses and to give them teaching or support'. She also considered that part of her clinical function was to do with the nursing philosophy. As she explained:

Each nurse has their own area of clinical responsibility – mine is 'making explicit the nursing team's philosophy, identifying the appropriate framework for practice, and ensuring that all staff understand the implications for practice'.

She related this to work she was undertaking on the development of a nursing model which she hoped would 'help the nurses to achieve direction', and to work she was doing on developing the care plans and redesigning the paperwork.

Owing to the 'collegiate' nature of the role, and the absence at that time of a ward sister, she and the senior nurse 'shared the clinical function . . . by working in parallel, by being equal partners'. In this respect, she described two areas of overlap with the senior nurse as 'monitoring and developing the quality and nature of nursing care' – she saw her role as 'going right down to the fundamentals and looking at what the nurses are doing, what they should be doing' – and 'ensuring that district policies are understood and adhered to, as any senior nurse would have to do'.

Staff development

Staff development meant similar activities for the five LPs. Thus Beth talked about 'working with individual staff to maximise their potential' and 'promoting the personal and professional growth of the team', and Ann similarly stressed both the individual growth, and through that, the development of nursing practice. Likewise, Ellen referred to 'facilitating the learning of the staff nurses' and 'working with the team leaders' to enhance their roles. She also talked a great deal about 'providing support for the nurses' as being part of the same aspect.

Both Charlotte and David referred to developing the staff as being important in the sense of developing nursing practice in the ward/unit and, for Charlotte, enhancing the role of the nurses and ensuring that all 'accept maximum responsibility within the bounds of their jobs'.

As well as notions of individual, team and nursing practice development, all saw the development of staff as necessary to the preparation of the clinical area prior to students arriving. In particular, Beth linked this with the preparation of staff nurse mentors for the undergraduate programme.

In terms of what they did to develop the staff, with Ann and Beth it was integral to their work on the ward. They hoped that whilst working alongside or in the same team as staff nurses, they would, as Beth said, 'gain from the way [they] cared for patients in general, or the ways [they] handled certain situations'. Similarly, Ann was trying to get her nurses, particularly the more junior ones, to 'have a more flexible approach to their work', and in the long term to 'develop them to make professional decisions about what's important and what's not'. In doing this, though, Ann described the problems and the tensions that arose when trying to combine looking after patients with being proactive in the development of her staff:

On a busy day, I tend to look after my patients ... [they] are the focus. And I just hope that I am working with two professional nurses who can cope with their own workload because my workload is more than I can cope with at that moment. I suppose in the quieter moments you're doing the staff development, to buck them up for the worst periods ... I suppose they are watching what you're doing ... I sometimes find that they are doing things that I do.

And further, she said: 'I feel this overwhelming desire to spend *more* time with my staff – to help them grow and develop and learn more about nursing practice, but the demands of the job preclude this.' In addition, both Ann and Beth spent time talking with staff about taking part in study days and other events that would help in their development.

Charlotte and David too did not strongly distinguish staff development from the range of activities they undertook in their time on the ward/unit. Development of staff was something that they considered happened in part through their normal interaction with the nurses and in part when nurses came and talked with them about events or activities that they were, or wished to be, involved in.

Ellen, on the other hand, engaged in a number of relatively discrete activities with the aim of 'facilitating the staff'. These included 'working on individual staff development programmes'; spending time every week with individuals to help them, for example, write an application form, or improve their interview technique; and, in conjunction with the senior nurse, spending a day with the team leaders to look at different issues. In addition, she 'provided support for staff nurses', when she was on the ward, something that she linked with staff development.

Management and administration

All of them considered management to be part of their role. For three, this was by virtue of them being senior sisters of a unit and 'sisters' for a ward, whereas for Ellen, who saw herself as a senior nurse and in a collegial relationship with the senior nurse for the unit, being a manager meant being in a shared role with the other person and having joint responsibilities. In fact, every aspect of the managerial function section of Ellen's job description was identified as overlapping with the senior nurse.

David's position was, however, more ambivalent. Whereas through choice he discussed some management issues with the senior nurse, and through necessity he acted up for her when she was on sick leave and after she had resigned, David did not see his role as being heavily involved with the management of the unit, but rather only in those matters that were directly related to staff.

For three of them (Ann, Beth and Charlotte), part of their job as managers was to manage or 'sort out' the budget, which was seen as part of the larger issue of managing resources. This entailed scrutinizing budget information, relating this to staffing and resources (e.g. supplies and equipment), making decisions about how their budget should be spent and what their staff skill mix should be, and sometimes, arguing the case for further resources. Neither David nor Ellen was a budget holder in their own right, though both had some involvement with it. For example, Ellen set up an educational fund to enable staff to have study days and attend conferences.

Another aspect was staffing. Whilst Ann, Beth and Charlotte were responsible for recruitment and selection of staff, and for the skill mix on their wards, Ellen shared these responsibilities with the senior nurse and David's role was very limited in this respect. The work involved monitoring staffing levels and grades, ascertaining when staff were likely to leave, organizing for advertisements of posts to be placed, interviewing and appointing staff.

Ann, Beth and David related such strategies as dependency studies (that is, working out the hours of nursing needed for individual patients and matching this to staff hours available) to reviewing the skill mix of the ward nursing staff. Beth explained that this was vital 'because when [she] took on the post as lecturer practitioner, the ward was under-resourced in terms of the nursing hours available'. Her aim was to be assured of sufficient resources, so that she could work and plan within her budget allocation.

For Ann, Beth and Charlotte, attending senior sisters' meetings and 'being on for the hospital' were part of their managerial function, whereas Ellen and David attended such meetings either by virtue of their status as senior nurses, or by negotiation with others.

Two of the five – Ann and Beth – talked separately about 'admin' (administration) as being an identifiable part of their role, in that Ann had special days she designated 'admin days', and Beth, 'flexi-days'. Ann saw the benefits of having such a day as 'being able to clear [her] desk, and get in contact with people'. For the other three, administration was referred to only as part of other aspects, such as working on the ward, or in relation to 'Poly' work.

Charlotte was involved in a range of similar activities, particularly to do with staffing and budgets, but these were normally embedded in days when she was on the ward. Ellen talked about 'doing admin' as part of other aspects, but she did distinguish between 'paperwork admin' (e.g. reading reports and the latest clinical learning environment audit; update information about the 'Poly' course and requests for references) and other admin, which was 'primarily people coming to see [her] to talk things through'. David only talked about administration as being a separate activity when he was acting up as senior nurse.

The five lecturer practitioners and the first year of research

To summarize the position at the end of the first year of the research for the five, a 'vignette' of each is presented.

Ann took up post as a lecturer practitioner one year prior to the start of the research, with many years' experience as a ward sister and nurse tutor, and a strong commitment to the philosophy of nursing and nurse education in the district. This, combined with her familiarity with the ward (she had previously worked there as a clinical practice development nurse), facilitated her understanding of what she felt the role was about, and provided her with a definite strategy of the developments she hoped to achieve, both for the job and for the clinical area. Working on the ward and developing practice were the paramount aspects of the role for her, and the ones on which she spent the most time. In fact, she described the development of her staff and, through them, nursing practice as one of the major achievements of the first stage of her job.

For her, working on the ward meant sometimes having a caseload – either as the primary nurse, though more usually as an associate nurse – or working with patients as needed. The reasons for this were both professional and personal. And as well as providing and developing good practice as a practitioner in her own right, she saw this work as being for the development of the ward as a whole and for the development of staff, the three aspects being integral to one another. As such, though she distinguished it as a separate entity in the way she conceived aspects of her job, for Ann, many elements of staff development were not in practice separated out from the day-to-day working on the ward. Thus, as she went about her work, she talked with and supported the nurses.

Much of her activity was related to her role as senior sister; for example, the management of the budget, issues to do with staffing, attendance at senior sisters' meeting, and 'being on for the hospital', though she saw the task of management as being an overarching concept that affected all the other aspects of her job, rather than being a separate part of it. Doing admin, however, was separated out in the sense of time allocation; she tried to have admin days during which the focus of her activity was responding to a range of different, mostly written items.

Ann saw an important part of her role as publicizing the role, either by talking to others nationally or by having people come to the ward. In line with her job description (written by herself), Ann accepted that part of her job was 'to prepare and contribute to the educational programme of nurses in relationship to the theory and practice of nursing'. However, at the beginning of this stage, Ann's involvement in this (described as 'Poly' work) was limited, though towards the end, the balance had shifted somewhat. Ann was excited by this, and could see 'all the hard work spent in developing clinical practice' coming to fruition, in the preparation for having undergraduate students placed in the clinical areas.

Beth's role was, in many ways, very similar to that of Ann. She too had a strong clinical and teaching background, primarily in surgical nursing, when she took up the post. Like Ann, when working clinically she was most usually an associate nurse, though occasionally had her own primary patients. She described the issue of practice being central to her whole job as 'critical' and as her 'hobby horse', and one that brought many benefits, professional and personal.

Staff development for Beth was also integral to working on the ward, or something she built into a flexi-day. She used the term 'management' especially in the context of managing people, such as staff appraisal, identifying strengths and experience, and career planning, and considered that in the first 18 months of her job she had focused very much on the management of people in the unit, because 'through them [she] was able to affect clinical practice'. Admin was considered as a separate activity, in as much as she had admin ('flexi') days, but was otherwise integral to other aspects. In common with Ann, she too believed in the importance of talking and writing about the job and exposing it to others interested in the plans and the reality.

Before September 1989, the balance of the job was far more in favour of developing the clinical areas and being in practice. She had a sense of being isolated, because lecturer practitioners were viewed as 'different from the rest [of the 'Poly' department]', but after this time, the commitment towards 'Poly' work, and the actual activities engaged in expanded. This was matched by her increased feeling of being part of the Polytechnic as well as part of service. She was aware of others seeing the job as 'huge and burdensome' whilst for her it was 'reasonable and interesting'.

Ellen had previously been a clinical teacher in the area in which she was appointed as lecturer practitioner. She had 'always been in favour' of the collegiate role, seeing the job as too big for one person to do justice to all the aspects.

She found the distinction made in the job description of clinical, educational and managerial functions helpful in terms of clarifying what she did or was accountable for, but not realistic in terms of how she achieved the different aspects, since many were integral or overlapping rather than separate. Conceptually she saw the job as a 'unified whole', with the different activities being component parts, all contributing to the whole. Critical to the achievement of the job was the notion of a partnership between her and the senior nurse, which needed to be worked out, but then reviewed at intervals.

Working clinically and supporting and working with other nurses was part of Ellen's way of 'developing standards of patient care', 'managing' and 'developing the clinical learning environment', all of which she saw as areas of her remit. Additional aspects of her accountability were budget planning, 'Poly' input, development generally and her own professional growth.

The way in which she fulfilled her role was by having separate phases or periods of time, during which she focused on particular activities, such as clinical work, developing the staff, planning, and so on. She spent a great deal of time 'reviewing her role' and articulating it to others. Further, in the absence of the senior nurse for three months she acted across, something which strengthened her conviction that aspects of the job, particularly the clinical and managerial responsibility, should be shared. Like Ann and Beth, the 'Poly' part of her work was increasing towards the latter part of the period.

David's role as a lecturer practitioner was different from the other four in two respects: first, he gradually took on the job of lecturer practitioner, spending only one day a week in the unit for about the first six months (i.e. from November 1988), and second, he retained his role as a tutor in the school of nursing (one he had held for the previous five years) for the rest of the time. This orientation, and the expectations it brought, had a considerable bearing on the way in which he conceived his role and what he actually did.

After the first six months, David was expected to be in the unit for half of the week, with the rest devoted to tutor or 'Poly' work. This was very much how he saw the job – as divided into two parts. However, the understanding of others about the unit work was sometimes at variance with David's, in that he saw the practitioner role as being about the development of clinical practice and the nurses on the ward, whereas others saw it as providing a clinical input (i.e. having a caseload and easing the staff shortages). This proved to be a tension in the job.

David made a distinction between 'Poly' work and tutor or school work in the other half of the job. Whilst he felt he should 'see the RGN students through', partly because of his previous tutor role, and partly since he was paid by the school, the amount of time this took up was problematic. Nevertheless, there was always a much more even proportion of the job spent in the two parts – service and education – than with the other four.

The role of David as manager was one of the aspects that contributed towards his decision to leave. During the first stage, the senior nurse – the manager of the unit – was frequently absent and David had to take on managerial responsibilities. This tended to detract from the successful undertaking of aspects of the lecturer practitioner role, especially the development of the nursing practice in the unit. When David was officially asked to act up as manager of the unit, following the retirement of the senior nurse, he did so in part to facilitate the role of lecturer practitioner, for, at the time, 'there seemed the possibility that it would become a unit headed up by a lecturer practitioner'. This did not happen and another senior nurse was appointed. David decide to resign the post for a mixture of reasons, including frustration at the lack of progress in the unit, lack of support in the module planning team, the general workload and the inability to find the time to prepare sufficiently for his degree exams, a long-held desire to leave the area and/or the profession, as well as other more personal reasons.

Charlotte took up post having been a clinical teacher with post-basic students, and she was keen to get back into clinical nursing 'in a sphere where [she] could influence change'. Her role as a lecturer practitioner was different from the others in that she was only accountable to the director of nursing service and not jointly paid by the health authority and the Polytechnic, though she did anticipate that eventually some proportion (possibly a quarter) would be paid for by the 'Poly'. Further, her job description was the original one that she had had when appointed, and this described primarily a senior nurse post with some lecturer practitioner duties. Therefore, she saw her job initially as that of a senior nurse, but with an understanding that she would be preparing the clinical area for the forthcoming students undertaking the elderly care module from September 1990. She anticipated, in the future, taking on some educational aspects of a lecturer practitioner's role, but not all. In a sense, she was a senior nurse with 'a lecturer practitioner part that included clinical teaching, but not "Poly" lecturing', and she described herself as 'a clinical lecturer practitioner'.

Further, she did not see herself as quite the same as the others in that she was previously a clinical teacher, rather than a tutor. She considered that the former was 'not a qualification for being a lecturer practitioner', but that it was necessary (for the 'Poly') to take on such people, particularly in elderly care, to 'get through the interim period when there are not enough people with the appropriate qualifications'. This had implications for the way she construed her job and the things that she did.

As a result of these two factors – the orientation of the job towards that of a senior nurse and the different qualification possessed from other lecturer practitioners – Charlotte described herself as 'not a standard lecturer practitioner'. As such, in general, she made no overt distinctions between management, practice and educational aspects of the job, but rather between types of activity, such as being involved in the elderly care module and attending lecturer practitioner meetings on the one hand, and preparing the clinical areas and developing the nurses and the information systems on the other. On any one day she could be involved in one or several of these and/or other activities.

The fact that she was not a standard lecturer practitioner made her feel at times to be 'in an ambivalent position'. She did not want to push too far on the lecturer practitioner side of her role (because of her officially sole accountability to the DNS and because of her background). But she considered that this in some ways was an unsatisfactory position to be in, and one that did not accurately reflect the reality of her situation – that in practice she was having to do the lecturer practitioner job.

In any case, she had reservations about the viability of combining management, practice, education and managing a budget in 'what is a huge job'. In relation to the undergraduate programme, there were many elements of uncertainty at that time, and it was a gradual process of people 'deciding what was needed and possible'. Part way through the period of observation, she was having problems in her dealings with a senior nurse manager. Despite considerable efforts on Charlotte's part, plus the involvement of others, the situation worsened and the problems seemed intractable. This had a severe effect on the way she conducted and felt about her job, consuming a good deal of her time and energy, and eventually led to her seeking other employment, and her subsequent resignation from the post in September 1990.

The four lecturer practitioners and the second stage

The four studied during the second stage were Ann, Beth, Ellen and Felicity. For all four, the job of lecturer practitioner remained complex and multi-faceted, and three of them – Ann, Beth and Ellen – continued to stress the 'integrated' and 'unified' nature of their roles.

However, Felicity talked about how initially she had not really seen her role as unified, and it was not until this stage that it became so. For her, this was in part a question of the reality of her responsibility for students, but it was also to do with the location of activities. Thus, as she said:

> I wasn't operating in a unified way before. Since the students have come here the role has changed completely – I'm on the ward for five days, I'm here all the time. It doesn't really come together until students hit your patch. I can see now how the bits fit together; ... the activities are unified with the ward and I do things with the students here – I'm on the ward, rather than spending half my time [in the Poly].

All four continued to have clinical activities as a critical part of their job. For three – Ann, Beth and Felicity – this still meant working regularly on the ward, usually as associate or team nurses, fitting in where needed and not normally being the co-ordinator for the shift. However, the pattern of their work was different from before, and they distinguished between term time and non-term time. Interestingly, whilst Beth considered that she worked more clinically out of term time, six days a fortnight compared with four days a fortnight in term time, Felicity described a higher input to the ward in term time, with 'the necessity to go outside the ward more at other times'. Ann distinguished between three phases – term time with students, term time without students (the last three weeks) and 'out of term' time. She tended to be on the ward more in term time when students were there, so that she could 'take the pressure off mentors' and enable them 'to be with their students'. Also, out of term time she had fewer other commitments, and she wanted to assure her ward staff that she was 'just a normal sister again ... and had time to spend with them'.

The pattern of working on the ward for Ann and Beth was determined, much more so than with Felicity, by the needs of the ward. For example, Beth spent more time working clinically when she had two primary patients to look after, and during one period when 'there were considerable difficulties on the ward with staffing'. Likewise, Ann worked 'practically five straight shifts a week' during one month 'because of the desperate shortage of staff', whereas during the following month she only did 'occasional shifts'. Such an obvious alteration in the balance of activities was not evident with Felicity when the ward was short staffed.

Ann and Felicity were much happier about their work on the ward than before. For Ann, it was a matter of feeling that she was coping better with the pressures of the job. Whilst unsure about the reasons for this, she made a suggestion, saying:

I'm not sure why I feel better about [the ward work] than at the beginning, but I seem to be able to do more with my time. And although the dependency figures indicate that the ward has actually been busier, it may be that I am thoroughly familiar with the situation and more realistic about what can be done.

Felicity, however, was more concerned about her ability to influence practice and the closeness of her relationship with the ward staff. In this respect, she linked her clinical role with the notion of where – physically – she was working. She talked about other people's uncertainty about her role in the clinical area, and the importance of 'having a high profile' in the early period, this meaning to Felicity actually 'being seen to be around'. Since initially she was 'so often off the ward', and staff did not know her well, she considered this to be problematic. But as this stage of her job, she was 'around the ward for five days' and therefore much more visible to the ward staff. Also she had 'negotiated to carry the level bleep' and so was on call to sort out unit problems. This felt more satisfactory to her.

Beth, it appears, had found the ward work more stressful at this time, but this was mainly to do with extraneous factors that were, in some senses, irrespective of her role as a lecturer practitioner. This included 'shortage of nurses of the right grade and experience, and the consequent tendency for them to rely on her more for decision-making than before', as well as her retaining some longer-term patients who had required a 'great deal of nursing' as her primary patients for several months. Nevertheless, she said that whilst before she had not considered the job to be 'too big' or 'burdensome' initially, she was much closer to believing that to be true, and was 'tired and irritable' because she was taking on too much.

Ann, Beth and Felicity were still involved with 'clinical projects', and developing clinical practice, though for Ann and Beth they were part of their 'normal' sister/senior sister role, and only Felicity singled clinical projects out as a separate activity from ward work.

All four continued to be involved in a range of activities aimed at the development of staff and all saw the preparation of mentors as an important part of the development of the staff nurses. Ann and Beth also referred to the need to develop the staff 'so that they are able to take on greater autonomy and responsibility within the ward', for without this 'it would be impossible for them [Ann and Beth], to achieve all that was necessary on the ward'. As Ann said:

I have my staff nurses doing a number of things such as preparing the off-duty, allocating students to mentors, overseeing the clinical learning environment, arranging an annual clinical learning audit, and attending to clinical nursing standards. This is the way we work on the ward, but also I simply wouldn't have the time to do it all myself.

Clearly this kind of situation was different for Ellen and Felicity because they did not have the managerial authority for the ward, though both distinguished those aspects that were to do with staff development and student learning as very much part of their brief. Felicity used three criteria – 'staff development', 'ward atmosphere' and 'resource implications' – when deciding on whether she should be involved. She said:

> If I can argue that it's to do with staff development for the ward [including orientation, selection and recruitment], or it's to do with harmony or anything that's going to affect the atmosphere on the ward [such as an unhappy nurse on the ward], or it's going to have major resource implications, which could be that the workload increases so that the nurses are stretched, then it's my role. For example, there have been discussions on a day case unit. I would see myself being involved in that because it may be a place we want to send students to. Also, if they hive off two or three of our nurses to go and run it, that's going to have an effect on the overall cover, the support you can give students as well as the effects on patient care.

In respect of both staff development and clinical development, during the early period of her job Felicity felt that she had achieved 'considerable progress ... against difficult odds', identifying the main impediment as the insufficient 'formal authority for policy-making in the [clinical] area and opportunity to respond to planned initiatives'. During the current period, she described certain movement which she related to her 'higher profile' on the ward and the improved clarity of her role.

Though Ellen was still involved in staff development, there were some changes in that her role was much more oriented to the unit at this stage, whereas before a particular ward had been her focus. This meant that she was 'relating to a much larger number of staff'. In addition, the nature of her relationship with staff of that ward changed because of the appointment of a ward sister, and the need for them to work out their mutual roles.

Whilst the other three talked about their role in supporting the ward staff as they went about their jobs, only Ellen referred specifically to the strategies adopted for staff support. This may well have been, as Ellen identified, due to the sensitive and stressful nature of the work in palliative care. Since the first stage, the nature of the staff support had changed. Before, the ward staff support group had been 'one of

[her] big involvements' and now she 'was pulling out', partly because of the new ward sister and partly because the staff felt that the group was not in itself sufficient. Therefore, Ellen was helping them with a broader strategy for staff support. Further, a critical aspect of Ellen's role now was 'the support of staff across the unit'. It took up a great deal of her time at this stage because two new parts to the unit – a pain unit and an Imperial Cancer Research Fund unit – were established during this period.

All were still involved in the range of activities that Ann and Beth described as 'part of being a senior nurse/ward sister', and that Ellen and Felicity saw as part of their managerial responsibilities 'within their collegial roles'. These included interviewing, selection, recruitment and induction of new staff. Felicity suggested that she was involved in such aspects in part because the calibre of the nurses recruited affected the learning environment and in part because 'it was important for [her] credibility [as a senior nurse]' and that 'if [she] did not exercise that kind of authority, then [she] was just a visitor to the ward'. For Ellen, this was very much part of her shared managerial role with the senior nurse.

The most noticeable change, in terms of both the amount of time and range of activities, was to be found in the education or 'Poly' aspect of their roles. This now included module planning, mentor support and development, contact with students, validation of learning contracts, moderation, teaching, being a professional tutor and attending meetings for all and, in addition for Beth, chairing an Assessment of Practice Group.

Being a lecturer practitioner at the third stage

The pattern of Ann, Beth and Felicity's lives was very similar to the previous stage in terms of the type of activities, but the balance of these was variable; the precise way in which they worked and their attitudes to the job had altered in some respects. Ellen's position was somewhat different in that she negotiated extra study leave and did not resume all aspects of her role until the Summer term.

Ann, Beth and Felicity continued to work on the ward, spending about the same amount of time in clinical activities and occupying the same kind of role. However, Ellen's clinically related activities – apart from the development of assessment and care planning on one ward which formed the research and dissertation for her course – were 'pared down to the minimum'.

All distinguished more overtly between term time and out-of-term-time. In term time, it was more difficult for the three to work complete shifts because their Polytechnic commitments had increased. As Ann said:

> During the term time with students, when I do an early shift I'm often gone by 2 pm because I've got to do a tutorial [with the students] or there's the seminars.

The busy-ness of the ward and the availability of staff with the right experience affected Ann and Beth less during this time. Ann had not done as much clinical work during the second term as normal. She explained that the amount she worked on the ward varied according to 'whether the ward needed her or not' and was 'driven' by this. If the ward was short of staff she would 'work five days a week', but during this period 'the staffing seemed so much better than in the early days' and so she was not needed as much.

That pattern pertained also for Beth in that working on the ward was in part dependent on the staffing. She explained that 'with good staffing levels, [she] could choose to absent [herself] for a week at a time to focus on other work'. This for her was one of the issues of the job and an implication of being the ward manager as well a lecturer practitioner, in that 'one does feel a lot of personal responsibility for the ward and uses oneself to fill in the holes when things are really bad'. In this respect, she talked about 'being at the whim of the staffing'. Conversely, Felicity did not feel the same sense of responsibility for ensuring that staffing was adequate, nor in filling the gaps. Indeed, there were three weeks at one point when, 'despite the busy-ness of the ward, because of moderation, Exam Board, and evaluation meetings, [she] had been unable to do anything more than put in a brief appearance'.

Ann, Beth and Felicity talked about problems stemming from their practice necessarily in some weeks being 'bitty' and 'lacking continuity'. For Ann in particular, her inability to work continuously with primary patients caused her 'some disappointment' because she enjoyed working in this way, and considered that this enabled her to 'act as an advanced practitioner'. Nevertheless, she considered that earlier she had given the ward staff 'a demonstration of good practice', that they were satisfied with her as a role model and she did teach them clinically.

All used the term 'credibility' much more and considered that 'being seen to be a competent practitioner', 'playing one's part in ward work', and 'having an influence over practice' had a vital bearing on this. Indeed, despite not being able to work clinically and only minimally in clinical related activities, Ellen said:

> The staff on Ward X know me well, they know I can do the work,

and ... therefore in their eyes I am credible. ... However, I do plan to go and work in [another part of the unit] next, and there should be a trade-off. They can introduce me to ... things like epidural anaesthesia and I might be able to help them teach their staff etc. In that way they will see what I have to offer clinically.

Credibility for the four was also related to their authority within practice. Ann and Beth felt their authority 'to be enhanced by being credible practitioners'. Ellen and Felicity were in collegiate managerial roles and initially had no automatic clinical responsibility. For them, having clinical credibility meant that others saw them as people to turn to for advice and guidance on clinical matters (in the broadest sense, not just in relation to individual patient care). For example, Felicity said: 'I find that ward staff are much more inclined to come and ask me what they should do about this, or how they should tackle that.'

All of them were engaged in staff development as before, and this was one of the aspects that Ellen had 'chosen to prioritize' during this period. However, three of them in particular talked about how the careful work in the past had resulted in a partial diminution of their roles in certain respects, in relation to both what they needed to do with staff as well as aspects of managing the wards. They all described it similarly, referring to such notions as being successful in what they set out to achieve, but making themselves redundant in some respects in the process. For example, Ann said that she felt she had in part 'worked [herself] out of a job because of the tremendously successful work in terms of staff development'. This had entailed

a lot of investment in terms of developing roles, clearly identifying them and then helping people to fit into those roles and to perform well in them ... the development of leadership.

Thus, she had ensured a 'really high standard of practice' on the ward, and ward staff who were capable of 'running the ward themselves'. Beth, too, considered that 'the ward did not need [her] as much as before because of getting good people into post and giving them the support they require'. In addition, Beth suggested that her role in relation to new staff was not as fundamental as before. This she attributed to the stronger ward ambience saying:

The same issues were around at this time because of new staff and their orientation and absorbing of the culture. But the culture [of the ward] is now much stronger [in terms of] what kind of nursing we operate, and it doesn't need me to tell them what it is, they pick it up through other cues.

Ellen, too, felt that her early work with ward staff had had implications. She explained:

> [Ward X] is doing very nicely now and I can't justify going down there as much. They are moving on in leaps and bounds. I'm effectively becoming more redundant, which I take as a measure of success of the role. We have other nurses doing what I was doing two to three years ago, and they are catching up so quickly, which is wonderful. Therefore my input [on that ward] is less.

Nevertheless, all of them still saw the importance of offering the staff support, even if not providing the same kind of leadership and direction as before. It appeared to be this aspect of support, exemplified by 'being around when the staff needed them', 'ensuring that they got the opportunities to go on study days' or 'popping down to the ward to see how they were, and/or having a cup of coffee with them', that typified their relationship with the ward staff at this stage.

The amount of time that Ann and Beth spent on administration had diminished for three main reasons. First, they shared a secretary with other lecturer practitioners and she had increasingly taken on aspects of administration. Second, they were becoming more efficient, thus reducing the time involved and, third, Ann was no longer responsible for the administration in relation to the second ward on her unit.

However, Ellen and Felicity's positions were different at this stage. Ellen's involvement in the senior management activities was pared down and she said that the senior nurse 'tried to not ask [her] to do anything during that period of time'. She and the senior nurse attempted

> to minimize her input on the planning and negotiations in relation to [two new clinical areas in the unit], but an enormous amount came up that the senior nurse could not carry on her own ... so [Ellen] did little bits, but not a lot, and the senior nurse was essentially co-ordinating the work.

Ellen explained that 'this was an area that [she] could not completely let go on because the future of the unit was at stake'. Further, during this period she 'abandoned all non-urgent meetings and dealt only with urgent mail, [she] did not take on anything new and shelved as much as possible'. However, the 'pile of papers to deal with during the summer was huge'. (This was exacerbated by an increase in the amount of 'service admin' overall because of resource management issues and the opening up of two new clinical areas within the unit.)

Perhaps the greatest change amongst the four occurred for Felicity. Under the new managerial and resource management arrangements for the paediatric services, she had become the Service Delivery Unit

(SDU) manager for her ward. This had a number of implications for her job. First, it helped clarify her role and that of the two other senior nurses with whom she worked closely. Second, it changed her managerial responsibility in relation to the ward; for example, she became the budget holder for her ward. Third, it increased the number of meetings she was required to attend. And fourth, whilst initially she found that the amount of service admin increased as her role 'became more comfortable', rather than feeling that she had to do everything herself, she was 'more able to hand things on to other people'. Felicity attributed her ability to devolve the work to others to the security she had accrued by now having the formal responsibility.

For Felicity, responsibility and authority were related to an official change in her managerial status. She considered that her position in respect of policy-making was much stronger, since she now had the authority, and the opportunity to respond to planned initiatives had improved greatly. This also helped in terms of her external image. As she said:

> I feel much clearer if I have to talk about my role at conferences etc. I don't have to worry about the fact that I am not the ward sister. I can say, 'I'm the SDU manager and I've got the budget responsibility and the education role' – and that makes sense to people.

The type of work that the four described as 'Poly work' or 'educational activities' was much the same as before, in that it included module planning, mentor preparation and development, direct contact with students, assessment of students, teaching, educational admin (considered as separate from service admin by Ellen and Felicity), and attendance at meetings. However, the nature of the activities varied, both from this period to the last and amongst the four.

The survey of lecturer practitioners

The survey was undertaken after the in-depth study of the six LPs had been completed. For the 55 LPs who responded (93% of all LPs in post excluding those already studied), it indicated that the range of activities was very similar to the six, but that the extent of involvement often varied. The nature of the practice role is of particular interest as are the satisfactions experienced. (The education role and the problems are discussed in subsequent chapters.)

The clinical or practice element of the role

First, the survey LPs were given a list of the kinds of activities engaged in by the six LPs and were asked to indicate which of the activities described the meaning of the practice element of their jobs to them. They could tick as many as were relevant. (The percentage of LPs indicating each is given in brackets.) Thus the 'practice' element of the job meant:

- working clinically, providing direct patient/client care (93%)
- developing clinical practice (e.g. through staff development and support, research, quality assurance and the like) (91%)
- working with or supporting others who actually give the care (78%)
- giving clinical advice (76%).

How the LPs actually fulfilled their clinical remit varied. (Figures in brackets represent percentages working in this way; more than one arrangement could be indicated.) Thus the way in which they worked clinically included:

- working as a primary nurse or with own caseload of patients or clients (for an average of two days a week) (42%)
- working as an associate nurse or team member (40%)
- occasionally working as a primary nurse or in similar role (15%)
- another arrangement (9%)
- working clinically in exceptional circumstances (e.g. when short-staffed) (9%).

A very small proportion (5%) said that they were rarely able to work clinically.

With respect to the pattern of their clinical work, the survey lecturer practitioners gave one answer only. Thus, the mode of clinical work was such that:

- they usually worked less clinically during term time (38%)
- the pattern was the same regardless of whether it was term time or not (38%)
- the clinical work had no discernible pattern (15%)
- they usually worked more clinically during term time (5%)
- another way of working was evident (4%).

The survey LPs were asked why they worked clinically and were given the choice of reasons that had been abstracted from the in-depth study. They could indicate more than one. Thus they worked clinically:

- for enjoyment (82%)
- to keep clinical skills up-to-date (80%)

- to demonstrate skills to students and nurses (73%)
- for clinical credibility (60%)
- because they were ... counted in the numbers/a member of the team (53%)
- because a clinical caseload was part of the job description (51%)
- because of staff shortages (44%)
- for other reasons (11%).

In relation to the feelings about the clinical aspect, 11% were very satisfied and 31% were quite satisfied with the clinical component, 22% were satisfied on the whole but would like to work more clinically, and 13% would like to work much more clinically. Conversely, three people (5%) felt they would like to work less clinically, and the feelings of eight (15%) were too complex to categorize as one of the above. (There was no response from two people, 3%).

Satisfactions of being a lecturer practitioner

The survey LPs were asked what they felt to be the satisfactions of the job and they could indicate up to three. Only two respondents felt that there were no satisfactions at all to be being a lecturer practitioner. The majority (53/55) gave responses that can be grouped into five overarching categories: relationships with others, primarily students, but also clinical staff, peers, managers and clients; developmental factors such as developing others, themselves, and clinical practice, as well as being innovative and facilitating changes; facets intrinsic to the role itself, for example, the combination of education and practice, the provision of patient and client care, and aspects such as teaching and research; characteristics of the role such as autonomy and authority, skills, expertise and credibility; and contextual and organizational aspects, such as being in a stimulating and supportive environment.

Relationships with others

By far the largest number of replies related to the students, with over half (32 or 58%) of all respondents making at least one reference to the satisfaction brought by the students. Typically, they mentioned the general points of: 'student contact', 'working with students', 'relationship with students'; 'having a close relationship with students throughout learning'; and 'the challenge posed by students'. They also made comparisons with their previous experience; for example:

'forming a stronger rapport with students'; and 'ensuring better continuity for students'.

There were several references to observing students grow and the part they as lecturer practitioners played in this process; for example: 'helping students develop their skills and attitudes and knowledge' and 'the opportunity to support students, and heighten their awareness and knowledge base of ... [nursing]'. Further, there were two references to the lecturer practitioners themselves gaining from this relationship by 'learning from students (as well as helping them)' and 'being valued by students'.

Three lecturer practitioners commented on the satisfaction gained from facilitating a pleasant experience for the students, as illustrated by the following: 'ensuring clinical practice and learning is a pleasant and exciting experience for students', 'sharing personal experiences with students helps students see the joy and pain of clinical practice' and 'students finding placements educational and enjoyable'.

Relationships with 'different groups' was another satisfaction. Six lecturer practitioners (11%) found these relationships a positive aspect of the job, describing them variously as 'involvement with students, mentors, staff, and clients in both settings', 'networking with students and mentors', 'being involved with patients and students' and 'learning from staff, colleagues and students'.

Development and change

Nearly a quarter of respondents (13 or 24%) claimed to gain satisfaction from 'developing others'. For example, when considering trained staff, some expressed this simply as: 'helping clinical staff to develop'. A few of the comments were rather more specific. Thus, 'facilitating others in the development of skills and knowledge', 'assisting nurses to develop their own ideas and theories' and 'seeing response from nurses who did not want to develop their own practice', were all viewed as positive aspects.

An identical proportion of lecturer practitioners (13 or 24%) referred to 'self-development and growth' as a positive aspect, for example: 'developing practice of myself', 'opportunity for personal professional development' and 'develop myself as thinking-doer'. Some mentioned the part played by being in practice as especially relevant – for example, having the 'opportunity to practise regularly and [thereby] develop own skills' and the 'personal competence acquired from practice'. One respondent considered that personal growth came both from clinical practice and education, and another talked about the chance to 'test new ground, and build [her] own confidence'.

A third aspect of development that received several mentions (11 or 20%) was that of 'developing nursing'. For some, this was a general comment, for example, 'implementing quality practice in [my] own and other clinical areas' and 'the freedom to explore nursing'. There was also a tendency to talk about the development of the clinical specialty, or a new service, hence the positive nature of 'clinical practice with clients with the responsibility to develop the specialty' and 'being involved in nursing development work, especially in a "cinderella" area'. In this respect, this type of response had a great deal in common with another category, that of 'raising the clinical profile'. Three lecturer practitioners considered this to bring satisfaction, as illustrated by the following: 'enhancing the profile of a disenfranchised area of nursing (i.e. learning disabilities)', 'raising awareness of the needs of diabetics' and the 'promotion of community nursing'.

The ability to 'change and innovate' was an attraction. Five respondents thought this was important, and valued: 'the challenge of the role', the fact that it was 'encouraging to see innovations in practice and to have this as a legitimate area of responsibility' of the role, and the 'excitement of a pioneering role', and more specifically 'challenging the old status quo and changing the role of the midwife'. Finally, three lecturer practitioners found the feeling that they were contributing towards 'shaping the future' to be positive. This was both in the sense of the students – 'shaping the next generation of nurses' – and for the profession – 'playing a key role in shaping nursing's future' and 'influencing the future of the profession'.

Aspects of the role

The satisfaction of being involved in or 'combining practice and education' in their roles was mentioned by 17 lecturer practitioners (31%). This was expressed either simply as 'having a clinical and education role' and 'having teaching and practice in the same job'. Or it was stated in a rather more complex way, for example, 'developing clinical practice and planning and delivering education for students' and 'having authority and responsibility for all aspects of the ward and an influential role in the education environment'.

Some gave apparent emphasis to either the practice or the education element and its relationship to the other, such as: 'combining nursing patients with other things, e.g. management, education' and 'having an educational job which lets me have patient contact'. In addition, one made a link between the two parts by talking about the satisfaction of 'being able to preach what [she] practised'. (In a connected category entitled 'links with practice', two lecturer practitioners were positive about them, saying that they valued 'knowing that what [they] teach students is directly relevant to practice', and 'having links with practice as a reality and not just a memory.')

Related to these comments, one talked about the positive nature of 'the legitimacy of giving direct patient care *and* education', another the satisfaction of 'influencing both practice and education', and a third referred to the 'academic' advantages – 'clinical practice combined with high level academic discussion that goes with the education aspect'. Another suggested that it was advantageous to 'have a foot in the two camps' at a time of uncertainty in relation to separate service and education roles.

Another satisfying aspect of the role was 'providing patient care' or 'having patient contact'. A total of nine lecturer practitioners (16%) gave this as one of their satisfactions, as exemplified by the following: 'retaining direct contact with patients', 'maintaining a clinical case-load' (three mentions), 'still dealing with practice issues', 'being able to work clinically', and 'practising my own clinical skills'. One tempered her comment by saying she found satisfying 'the contact with patients and clinical areas without [having] managerial responsibility'. Related to this category was that of 'achieving standards', with one respondent suggesting that 'encouraging and seeing high standards of patient care' was a positive aspect of her role.

A few respondents highlighted other aspects of their job. For example, four said they found 'teaching' satisfying – 'teaching and supporting students', 'teaching extra subjects I enjoy' and simply the 'chance to teach'. Two respondents mentioned 'research' – 'having a recognized research element' and 'being able to pursue professional interests, especially research'.

Characteristics of the role

A further important category, with eight lecturer practitioners (15%) giving it as a positive factor, was the 'autonomy' afforded by the job. Three actually used the term 'autonomy', whereas others described it as 'being able to set my own priorities', 'the freedom to plan work myself', 'the freedom to take role where I want to', 'the independence of the role', 'being my own boss' and 'being my own manager'. One distinguished between 'professional and personal autonomy' and another referred to 'the autonomy and authority in practice'.

The 'diversity' or variety of the role was mentioned. Seven respondents (13%) suggested that the 'diversity' and 'the variety of activities' was a positive aspect, and as one said, 'you never get bored because every day can be different'.

A few mentioned the personal benefits of the role. For example, four found the ability to use their 'skills and expertise' satisfying as exemplified by the following: 'having abilities in three interdependent areas', 'using management, education and clinical skills', 'being able to practise as an expert practitioner' and 'maintaining clinical expertise'. This last comment is similar to another type of response, whereby two people mentioned their 'credibility' and 'being recognized as expert in the clinical area as well as a teacher'. There appears to be a connection between these facets and another mentioned by two lecturer practitioners – that of the ability to 'keep up-to-date' and 'being supported to [do so]'.

Context

Five lecturer practitioners found the 'stimulating environment' satisfying, describing it as 'working in a stimulating education environment', 'being in contact with dedicated and bright colleagues', 'the regular contact with others' stimulating brains' and the 'exposure to challenge and debate'. One talked about the benefit of 'clinical practice combined with high level academic discussion'. Three lecturer practitioners talked about the satisfaction of the 'supportive environment', for example, 'the support of colleagues', 'supportive line managers' and 'the support and belonging to a group other than the clinical team'.

Finally, as mentioned before, though the research concentrated on the views of the lecturer practitioners themselves, the interview study of nursing staff gave an indication of what these people saw as the LP role. There were four LPs still in post at the time of the study of other people's perspectives. Thus, what follows are the views of mentors and team leaders, students and managers who worked with Ann, Beth, Ellen and Felicity.

Views of mentors and team leaders about the role

Most often the LP job was described as having three main facets, with the boundaries being somewhat hazy: education ('the LP part', 'the educator', 'the role with students'); the ward work ('being a ward sister', 'doing clinical work', 'being a team member/team leader', 'working clinically') and management ('being a senior nurse', 'being on for the hospital', 'the unit responsibilities'). Other aspects of the role were described separately, such as research, talking (nationally) about the role and 'attending meetings' (e.g. of national groups). These additional activities were not considered to be major parts of the roles, but were mainly mentioned in relation to the multi-faceted, pressurized nature of the job (for example: 'and on top of all that she's expected to do research'; 'in addition, because of her high profile, she gets asked to take part in groups and speak nationally').

Several felt that the role both of their lecturer practitioner, and of lecturer practitioners in general, had not initially been clear, and a few considered that it was still not *very* clear to them, and especially not to other nurses and students. Suggestions were made about its clarification, including making job descriptions more available and publicizing the job more widely.

What the lecturer practitioners were described as doing in reality varied across the four, but there were some commonalities. In particular, there was a high level of agreement over their 'strong educational role'. (The detail of what they thought this entailed is included in the next chapter.) In terms of the differences found within the group, these occurred mainly in relation to the aspects of the job other than education. The first of these was clinical work. Whilst three of the lecturer practitioners were deemed to 'work clinically on the ward', what this actually entailed was talked about in different ways. For example, in respect of two of them (Ann and Beth) it was seen more as an integral part of the job, and something that was expected of them, whereas with the third (Felicity) it only occurred 'when students were around on the wards', though one respondent mentioned that Felicity helped out, albeit infrequently, when the ward was very busy. The pattern of Ann and Beth's clinical work was variously described by respondents; for example, some said it was about two or even three shifts a week, others felt it was less frequent. Several pointed out that it varied according to whether it was term time, and which part of the term. Their roles were also described differently:

> She was a team leader most of the time because we had lost one of the F Grades; . . . I think the role suffered because of it [Beth];

> she's an associate nurse rather than a primary nurse, helping out in the team that most needs her [Ann and Beth];

> she likes to have/she does have one or two primary patients that she sees through [Ann and Beth].

In general, the fact that two of them in particular practised clinically was felt to be an important and necessary part of the role. A number of reasons were given for this. They included the notions that: it was a *sine qua non* of the role ('she wouldn't be a true LP if she didn't practise regularly'); it had value in keeping the lecturer practitioner in touch and up-to-date and thus able to talk knowledgeably to students about practice ('it must be better for the students because the person who is lecturing to them knows what it's really like on the ground'); it was important for other staff on the ward to see an advanced practitioner in action ('I've learnt a lot from seeing how she goes about things'); and it was deemed to bring personal satisfaction to the lecturer practitioners themselves. However, some mentioned problems in relation to it. For example, that of availability ('she is busy with other things during term time especially at the beginning and end'); continuity ('very often she comes on on an "early" [shift] but has to go off to a meeting in the Poly in the afternoon'), and the personal frustration experienced by lecturer practitioners when they could not work clinically as much as they would have liked. One respondent considered that her lecturer practitioner should be 'less involved with other things' and should spend more time working clinically and 'being around for the students' as she had expected her to be. Conversely, none of the respondents in relation to Felicity and Ellen considered that they should work more clinically.

Indeed, Ellen was not seen in the same ways as the others as having a clinical role. As one said, 'as I see it, her job is to ensure the educational needs of the people in the Unit – nurses and students', and another, 'Ellen is education'. This was not, however, seen as a problem since 'as long as she is in touch with what is going on in the ward, her job is to be there for the students and as a support for us, rather than actually giving hands-on care'. Another said, 'with all the other things she has to do, it would be unrealistic to expect her to spend more time working with patients'. And a third suggested, 'I know she would like to spend more time in practice but that is too hard to do because of her other commitments'.

A second aspect, described variously, was that of management. Two (Ann and Beth) were recognized as having a major managerial component to their roles by virtue of being ward sister and senior nurse, which entailed amongst other things 'managing the financial aspects, the budget', 'doing appraisals, interviewing', 'attending senior sisters' meetings' and 'being on for the hospital'. Nevertheless, most stressed that this sister role was different from a 'normal' sister's role. The following comment was typical:

> I suppose she fulfilled the notion of the sister's role and being there as a senior nurse to support the rest of the ward team. But a lot of her responsibilities that maybe would have been part of the traditional sister role were devolved down through the ward team.

Felicity, too, was recognized as having a management role, though this was felt to be clearer at a senior sister level. The ward management role was less obvious and did not concur with everyone's expectations. As one said:

> The thing that surprised me was how much of the ward management she's taken on, or has been forced to take on because of outside influences, taking into account that we have also got a ward sister.

Although, 'as a result of meetings between the sister and the senior staff nurse' and through changes in service management, Felicity's responsibilities, and how these dovetailed with the others on the ward, had become more evident, there was still some haziness about her role:

> We still find that there is a bit of confusion over where the sister's job finishes and the LP job starts. There is that overlap with a G grade on the ward. Having talked to some other nurses who haven't got a sister it's much more defined. It's difficult to define when there is a ward sister, a senior staff nurse *and* a lecturer practitioner. The newer staff nurses are not sure whether they should be going to the sister or the lecturer practitioner.

Respondents were very unforthcoming about Ellen's management role, especially in relation to the senior nurse. As one said, 'I am not sure where [the senior nurse's] management role stops and Ellen's starts, but I do know Ellen is more on the education side of things', but there was little mention of her managerial role from the others.

The views of students

In considering the nature of the role, students first and foremost talked about their experience with the lecturer practitioner on the ward. In this respect, they saw the role of the lecturer practitioner as 'helping to lay down what [they] were going to do for that module', 'being responsible for marking the learning contract', and 'being available should they have any problems that are to do with the module', or 'problems that the mentor can't deal with'.

In addition, all were engaged in some kind of interaction with the lecturer practitioner during the module, but the nature of this was dependent upon the module and the lecturer practitioner. Thus, for example, Beth's students talked about the student-led seminars whereby Beth 'took a back seat ... but asked questions to make you think, and gave you ideas on literature'. Ann's students mentioned 'a weekly gathering, called something like "the stress group"' which Ann facilitated, and the purpose was 'to have time to come together and talk about experiences and how [the students] were responding to them, to share anecdotes' and for Ann to 'provide reassurance that these [occurrences] were not peculiar'. Similarly, Ellen ran a 'support group' which she 'led initially, then facilitated'. For one of the students, this proved to be the main contact she had with Ellen, and an opportunity for 'going over the learning contract' after the meeting. One of Felicity's students was also her mentee and thus it was acknowledged that her experience of Felicity was not necessarily typical. However, the main aspect that was identified was 'a weekly reflection session' where the main purpose was 'to think in terms of the things that could go on the learning contract'.

Apart from student-related activities, and the fact that most mentioned that their lecturer practitioner was module leader, all were aware that the lecturer practitioner had a clinical involvement. With respect to Ellen, this was described as 'doing things with the nurses on the ward' rather than 'actually providing hands-on care'. However, apart from one student, most were unclear as to the exact nature of the clinical work; typically they saw the lecturer practitioner working shifts or knew that they did work on the ward, but they were unaware of the details. In terms of the differences, the students of two of the lecturer practitioners (Ann and Beth) were aware that they were sisters and 'did managerial things', but one relating to Felicity said that she was surprised that she was not a manager when she had been led to believe otherwise. Ellen's student made no mention of this aspect of the role. Further, several said that whilst they 'did not really know what else the lecturer practitioner did in the Poly', they were thought to be involved in 'numerous meetings', 'teaching on other modules' and 'doing presentations'.

The views of service managers

The service managers were not such a homogeneous group as the others in that two worked with one lecturer practitioner, one with another and the fourth with three of the lecturer practitioners. Further, they operated at different levels – one was a ward sister, two were senior nurses and one was a director of nursing services (DNS). This heterogeneity was reflected in their often quite different responses, which for three of them were related almost entirely to their own lecturer practitioner, and in the fourth instance was much more generalized. Nevertheless, as predicted, when asked about the role of their lecturer practitioner(s), two of them talked about the management aspects first, with the DNS making a distinction between the 'two different models occupied by the three lecturer practitioners'.

Of the other two, one stressed the emphasis of Ellen's role as on education ('I see her remit as being very much education, particularly for students but trained staff as well'), and on the consequent complementarity between her role as senior nurse and that of Ellen as LP. However, this respondent also made a distinction between her role as 'more to do with the economic side of things' and Ellen's as to do essentially with 'clinical management', by which she meant 'introducing something new in the clinical setting and facilitating someone else's ideas to innovate clinically in the ward'. The fourth talked about the distinction between her role as ward sister and manager, and Ellen as being 'a resource to the ward . . ., a source of support . . ., a help when a member of ward staff needs further information or advice, and a provider of tutorials for ward staff'.

Conclusion

Lecturer practitioners can clearly be viewed as having complex jobs, which, in the case of the six LPs, were seen to move through stages with an initial concentration on the development of their practice areas and the nursing staff with whom they were associated. Subsequently the emphasis on educationally oriented activities was increased, albeit alongside their – at times modified – practice function. The study of the LPs over the three years shed light on the way in which they developed their roles, and tackled the issues arising.

There were many similarities between the roles of the six LPs and those in the survey, especially in respect of the general principles underpinning them, the types of activities they engaged in, the attitudes expressed and the satisfactions gained. In addition, those people with whom the remaining four LPs from the in-depth study worked tended to have a realistic understanding of the role and, in general, to be supportive of it.

Chapter 5

Lecturer practitioners and student learning

As indicated in previous chapters, a major part of the role of all lecturer practitioners was the education aspect. This became a particular focus of the research, especially in respect of how the lecturer practitioners facilitated and ensured student learning. The questions posed by the research were: what understanding do lecturer practitioners have of their role in relation to students' learning; what do they do in practice to achieve students' learning; what are the problems/challenges related to this; and what distinctions are made between the roles of lecturer practitioner, mentor and lecturer? This chapter is devoted to illuminating the answers, first in respect of the six lecturer practitioners, then in relation to the survey lecturer practitioners. Finally, the views of mentors and team leaders, students and educators are elucidated.

The role at the early stage

The six LPs anticipated having limited direct contact with (undergraduate) students because the students were neither spending a great deal of time on their wards in their first year, nor were the lecturer practitioners greatly involved in teaching on the theoretical modules. Rather, four saw the 'education' aspect of their role as in some sense being about preparing for the students who would be in practice modules in their clinical areas in the second year. However, the approaches taken by the four varied.

Ann and Beth were similar in that they both concentrated on the development of their wards, and saw their 'main contribution to the Poly' at that stage as the development of a clinical area, including staff, that would be appropriate for students. For Felicity, 'developing the learning environment' entailed ensuring that the ward had up-to-date resources and books, and identifying and preparing mentors. Similarly, Ellen focused on staff development as 'an important preparation' for students, and she too attempted to improve 'learning resources' on the ward, both for the benefit of staff and future students.

Related to this clinical development work was the selection and preparation of mentors. All but Charlotte saw this as an important aspect of their work, and they appeared to consider that much of the teaching of students would be undertaken by other people, even at this early stage.

Only Ann and Beth were involved in planning and running seminars with the undergraduate students – though David did have substantial responsibilities for the teaching of RGN students. All, apart from Charlotte, were professional tutors to undergraduate students.

The sole activity described as 'Poly work', 'education' or even 'teaching' (using the term generically) that *all* six were involved in was planning the practice modules. It was through engagement in this that two of them (Ann and Beth) felt that they began to develop their identity as 'real lecturers', and they made the links between this opportunity for curriculum development and the direct influencing of student learning in the practice settings.

Thus, in conclusion, it appears that all (except David) were deliberately spending less (or much less) than 50% of their time on aspects referred to as educational, and that the main rationale and reality was the need to focus on clinical and staff development and, through this, the enhancement of the clinical areas for student learning. Further, there was a recognition of the part to be played by other people, i.e. mentors in teaching the students, and mentor selection and preparation was an important facet of the lecturer practitioner's role. Little or no time was spent in running seminars for, or in face-to-face teaching of, undergraduate students. Apart from a few observational visits of undergraduate students to some of their wards, the only direct contact lecturer practitioners had with these students at this stage was as their professional tutor.

Student learning in the second and third stages

All four had a broad conception of their educative function which was not restricted to direct contact with students, and which included module planning, mentor preparation and support, being a profes- sional tutor, and attendance at meetings. Direct contact was made with students by: helping students reflect on practice; conducting tutorials; running support groups; having meetings with students; working with or alongside students; being in the clinical area; assessing students;

and actually being a mentor, though the extent to which the four engaged in some of these activities varied greatly.

All considered that it was important to help the students to reflect on their practice, since they believed that learning was achieved in this way and the notion of learning through reflection underpinned the course. However, the way the four went about this was different. All used the discussions that took place for assessing the learning contract for this purpose, and Beth mainly concentrated on that process both to encourage and to assess the level of student reflection. In addition, she expected the mentors to be the main people with whom students reflected. She did not use particular planned strategies, preferring to work 'on an *ad hoc* basis', first judging how mentors worked with the students.

Likewise, Ellen did not have a particular approach, although she did use support group meetings 'to encourage reflection'. On the other hand, both Ann and Felicity actually held 'reflective sessions'. For example, Felicity had small meetings occasionally at the end of the day when students were on the ward. She considered that as well as giving all the students access to her, they allowed the students to 'reflect on their observations and practice' during the day. She saw the purpose of the sessions as the opportunity to 'talk things through, to make sense of what has happened and to relieve stress'. Ann described hers as small group 'debriefing sessions' based on story-telling about practice situations. Yet though she believed the sessions to be 'phenomenally useful' in that they provided stories or exemplars for the students to put into their contract, she was disappointed about the 'variable attendance' and the fact that clearly students did not agree with her view about their importance. From her descriptions, in these sessions it appears Ann tried to use her contextual knowledge of the ward and the instances that were cited.

Only one – Ann – held what she described as individual 'tutorials' with students, though all four made time to see students on an individual basis at the student's request. In terms of attendance at tutorials, however, Ann made a distinction between the weaker, average and stronger students. She said:

I do quite different things depending on the particular student. With a very weak student, the first tutorial was helping her get the work done from her last module. Then I needed to talk to her about clinical skills, how she was managing on the ward. Otherwise the purpose is to help the students to plan how they are going to manage the work they have do for the module. But for very bright students, I do not expect them to come to tutorials, because they cope and are learning independently. Then all I do for them is to be there so that they can use me in whatever way they want.

One of the four – Ellen – ran weekly support groups along with other lecturer practitioners for the students, the purpose of which was 'to offer the students a guarantee to see the LP to discuss whatever they wanted to discuss' as well as 'to contribute to the students learning, by helping them reflect'. Each of the groups operated 'according to its own ground rules'. The feedback from Ellen's group was that the majority of students found it a useful forum 'to share ideas and to discuss problems' in part because, as Ellen felt, 'the LP was able to stand back and see the situation in a broader context'.

Two of the four – Ann and Beth – instituted meetings with the students about half-way through the clinical placements, in order to get the students to say how they were getting on with the completion of their learning contracts. Beth suggested that she did this in part for the benefit of the students and in part for the mentors, saying:

> I did it so that the students would not be tempted to leave the completion of the learning contract until the end of the module as had happened with some students in the past, but also because last term the students didn't get the contracts in front of the mentors' eyes until the very end of term, and then the mentors couldn't remember some of the things that the students were describing.

During these meetings, students often raised other issues, such as the case study that they had to present. In addition, students came to see Ann, Beth and Felicity about their seminar presentations. Although the lecturer practitioners saw the purpose of these occasions as mainly to give students advice, and thus as learning opportunities for them, they were related to the process of assessment in that learning contracts, case studies and the seminars were all means of assessing the students.

The opportunity to work with or alongside students and being in the clinical area for the students appeared to be closely linked, and important aspects of the role for three out of the four. By the third stage, although she perceived it to be the role of the lecturer practitioner, Ellen specifically mentioned the impossibility of 'offering a one-to-one [relationship], either working alongside or being a role model for students', because of the number of students, the time constraints and primarily the fact that she was responsible for students in clinical areas other than her own. However, the other three felt that on an *ad hoc* basis they were always aware of the students when they (the lecturer practitioners) were working on the ward. For example, Beth's situation was typical of the three. She 'saw the students quite a bit in practice, working alongside their mentors and their patients' and felt that there might be situations where the student was unsure of what to do. She said:

> If I'm working on the ward I notice what students are up to; if I see one looking as though she's struggling I might ask her a couple of questions just in passing to get her to think more about what she was doing.

Beth was especially likely to talk to students if their mentor or the nurse they were working with was unavailable.

> There are situations where the students don't know where to turn next. For example, they may have learnt a number of skills in relation to individual patients, but when faced with a larger number, all demanding attention, they are not sure how to prioritize their work. If their mentor or the nurse they're working with isn't immediately to hand they would probably ask me. Or I would say 'what's on you mind at the moment' and encourage them to articulate the dilemma they're in, and help them work out what their options are.

Also, she said it was 'quite common', whilst she was working on the ward, to talk with students about patient care issues, or they might want some clinical information or advice. Similarly, Ann described situations, especially at weekends or when the mentor was not present, where she worked parts of shifts with students, either because she felt they needed support or because they requested it. Likewise, Felicity said: 'If the mentor is on night duty and the student wants to get cracking on the ward, I'll suggest they come and work alongside me for a couple of shifts'. In this instance, she described herself as a 'kind of co-mentor'.

In talking about their role in the clinical setting, Ann and Beth specifically referred to clinical teaching, with both making the point that they were not teaching clinically in the 'traditional' way, and describing what they actually did. Thus, Beth suggested:

> I'm not really involved in typical clinical teaching as in the old way. I'm not there showing them how to do things or working alongside as a euphemism for 'learning by Nellie'. It's actually only picking up with them where I'm an appropriate resource. Most of the time, their resource is their mentor or their patient and they're quite happy working independently.

And Ann said:

> As far as I'm concerned, clinical teaching is you working with the

student and supervising them and helping them to reflect etc. There's no way that a lecturer practitioner with five students could do that for all five. But as the students tend to work in teams – and quite often the day that they come the mentor isn't there – I might work with them as a member of the team. So, if ever I do teach clinically that's how I do it.

Being a mentor

The only one of the four who acted as a mentor during the third stage was Felicity. She considered that it was 'useful, if not essential [for lecturer practitioners] to have a go at mentoring, just to feel what it's like for mentors', but that she would not normally mentor because she 'wanted the staff nurses to have regular mentorship experience'. Further, in terms of the practicalities of her being a mentor, Felicity said that whilst she did not have the problem of having to co-ordinate the ward as well, there were other issues, such as being interrupted by phone calls.

Ellen had been a mentor once in the second stage, but neither Ann nor Beth had acted in this capacity, and neither saw it as the appropriate role for the lecturer practitioner. Beth argued this on the basis of practicalities and level of skill saying:

I don't think [lecturer practitioners] are there to work with students. Mentors are more than capable of doing that. It's a level of skill that should be in an E or D grade qualified nurse. I don't think it needs to be a highly qualified lecturer practitioner doing it because a) pragmatically it's not on and b) it's a waste of lecturer practitioner skills.

Beth suggested that this belief existed from the beginning, but that the stance had been confirmed for her during this stage:

I think I got an inkling that I wouldn't be able to do it all myself when I realized the numbers, and when we were in module planning. We talked about seven or eight students [per lecturer practitioner], and I thought then there's not going to be enough time to do that with each of them, and that it was going to have to be working through other people.

Validation of the students' learning contracts

The validation of the students' learning contracts formed the main and, for Ellen in the final stage, the only form of assessment of students during the clinical placements. A typical example from Ann serves to illustrate the pattern encountered with the LPs. Usually in the last week of the placement, the student and mentor met with Ann. She read the competencies and the student's 'reflection' on how he or she had achieved them, and asked for elaboration on the evidence of achievement, either from the student or the mentor. She often praised the student or she suggested to them that other competencies could also be covered by the information given, or that further data should be included to substantiate claims made. In that case, she gave the student the option of writing more later and adding to the learning contract afterwards.

She asked questions which appeared to be testing the student's attitudes and knowledge, including that gained in other modules. Ann tried 'to encourage the student to think more broadly and deeply' as she 'wanted to see how [the student] achieved the competence, and by asking questions, how much she knew. If she answered well, [she] wanted to push her even further'.

The meeting lasted at least an hour. Towards the end she asked the student and then the mentor what grade they felt the student should have. The student usually suggested a grade, albeit with encouragement, but if not, Ann said that either she would offer a view or ask the mentor for a view first. If the decision was not clearcut, and there was lack of agreement about the mark, Ann talked about it further, giving her reasons for a grade, and asking the mentor and student for theirs. In this instance, Ann felt that she 'had to be sure of the arguments since [she] had to justify the mark to the Exam Board'. She explained that the lecturer practitioner was responsible ultimately for the assignment of the grade, but that she used a process whereby the student was involved in self-assessment, and the mentor provided the detailed validation of the 'evidence' because she had worked most closely with the student. At the end of this process, they had a discussion about the competencies that were outstanding to be achieved in the next placement.

There were a number of small variations in this procedure with the other three. For example, typically, when Beth marked the learning contract one of the things that she talked about was whether the work 'showed movement' from the beginning of the module placement. In addition, she asked the student to tease out an example that the three of them could consider together, to examine the relationship between the competency achieved and the reflection. In this, Beth saw her role as helping the mentor as much as the student. As she said:

Some mentors are very able themselves at reflecting and don't need any support from the lecturer practitioner, but those who are not good at it need the lecturer practitioner to ask those questions of the student. If they don't, the student [suffers because] she is not getting any guidance on reflection. This is where the lecturer practitioner comes in.

In this respect, she considered that the three-way meetings were a good opportunity for them to 'learn together'. This point was confirmed by Felicity, who similarly said that the meetings were

a good opportunity to see where the mentor was at in terms of helping the student to reflect, and then to help the mentor to see how she could take the situation and reflect more on it.

One of the problems that Ellen found with the contracts, which she knew to be shared by others, was that the students tended to 'write them up the night before', whereas she wanted to 'get across the message' that it should be a working document. Within the validation itself, she said she found it helpful

to go through the grading criteria and to get the student to pull out their strengths and weaknesses in relation to these. This then made it easier for the student to identify which grade she was at.

In considering this procedure a number of key points emerge. First, all four appeared to use the validation of the contract as an opportunity for more than assessment. For example, it 'gave LPs the chance to encourage [students] to reflect on their practice', and was a way in which the lecturer practitioner 'brought theory and practice together'.

Second, it illustrated both the differences between the lecturer practitioner and the mentor, but conversely served to indicate the lack of clarity about and between the roles. For example, Felicity made the following overall distinction in the validation process whereby

the students are self-assessing their own competence, the mentor is validating that and the lecturer practitioner is looking at the academic level of reflection.

This appeared to be confirmed by Ann and Beth in a general sense, though in practice the process was more complex. Observed examples of Beth illustrated some of the possible distinctions between the roles of herself and the mentor. In these, the mentor in the main talked about her personal knowledge of working closely with the student – often pointing out aspects that the student had not included in the contract – and she referred to how (in her belief) the student was or was not achieving the competencies. Beth, on the other hand, looked 'more globally' at the contract. She picked up on examples given by the student 'to test out their knowledge', commented on the 'level of reflection' and indicated where the student could improve.

However, other observed and discussed examples – of Beth and the other three – showed nuances and variations. For example, the mentor was often, but not always, present, and had usually, though not always, indicated on the contract that the student had done what they said they had done. The student was normally asked what grade they would give themselves, and this was usually checked out with the mentor. But the lecturer practitioner was 'the person who decided finally upon the actual grade', and the extent to which it was influenced by the student and mentor, or the degree to which the mark was truly an agreed mark between the three, was variable. Indeed, all four acknowledged that they were judging far more than the adequacy and level of reflection and were, for example, testing the student's knowledge and understanding, challenging, asking questions and making suggestions to the student as well as getting the student to justify why they should be awarded a certain grade.

The variability of practice and lack of absolute clarity was deemed by Beth to be in part due to the novelty of the procedure, and to other factors such as the level of knowledge of the lecturer practitioner of the student. When responding to the researcher's account of it, she said how she was 'struck by an apparent method which [she believed] actually reflected what [she] did', though she said it had 'emerged out of personal experience' and she had never thought of it before as a 'conscious process'.

Third, there were issues arising in the validation that affected how the four felt about the task and how they went about it. There were two which were common to all, closely interlinked and raised by lecturer practitioners and students alike. On the one hand, there was the consideration about 'reflection on practice' – what it was and whether and how students learnt from such a process – and on the other hand, there was the nature of the relationship between reflection and the competence to practise as nurses.

The emphasis on learning through reflection was not only evident in the validation, but throughout the students' clinical placements and within other forums. However, as a notion it became more overt during the validation and was a topic of discussion and debate between lecturer practitioners, mentors and students. Although all four argued that they had both an understanding of what it meant and beliefs about it, it was still something that was new and that needed 'not to be taken for granted'. Typically, Ann, when responding to a question about learning nursing though reflection, made a distinction between 'reflection' and 'description' and acknowledged the lack of surety about it. She said:

I'm utterly convinced ... that good students can learn through reflection. I think the poorer students have great difficulty and they continue to just describe what's going on. But at least they are noticing what's going on. I think without the reflection they would never click at all. So I think its a good method of learning and you can certainly do it, but as with all things, it isn't a panacea. It's not going to make poor students good. Yet it's something that we are still not absolutely sure what it means in practice, and we need to do more work on it.

Felicity referred to 'talking things through and making sense of what happened', but what actually constituted 'reflection' and the exact nature of the learning occurring from it remained elusive to the four.

The nature of the relationship between the 'ability to reflect', the learning contract itself, and competence to nurse was also an issue that all explored. During an observation of Beth, one of the students said that she did not feel the contract fairly reflected her practice, but rather the ability to write a good contract. In interview, Beth contradicted this by saying:

On the whole I feel that the contracts do reflect practice. It is usually the weaker students who raise this objection. Also, undergraduates need to be able to articulate what nursing is about.

Similarly, Ann was concerned about students who argued they were good in practice, but were unable to express this in the contract. She explained:

They are now saying things to me like 'I'm good in practice, I just can't write it on a contract'. Well, I don't buy that. They have to be able to articulate what it is they do. That's part of being an undergraduate nurse. If they can't start developing that now, then they're not going to get good grades for their clinical practice.

And Felicity, too, disputed it as follows, saying:

The main time I have heard that said is by the weaker students who maybe think they are good in practice and then feel they are not getting the grades because they're not reflecting very well. But my feeling is that they are probably not performing at that level of practice. I don't really see that you can separate the two things. I think the ability to articulate on paper what you are doing in practice has to be there.

In addition, two of the four were concerned that the preparation of the learning contracts and the validation process were still problematic and in need of development, for a number of reasons. For example, mentors were not 'validating' all the actions of students, students were not writing the contract throughout their placements, and some lecturer practitioners were inexperienced in the use of learning contracts.

Comparison of role with mentors and lecturers

All four distinguished their roles from that of the mentor in terms of two main aspects – first, the differences in skills and knowledge, and second, what the two roles entailed. In relation to the first, Ann talked about her wider knowledge and skills in many respects saying:

> I am eminently better at coaching students, at helping them to reflect. My knowledge of nursing theory is so much greater. I'm much better read, I understand how people learn. I'm an experienced teacher; I've got so much more.

Felicity also talked about knowledge and skills in a similar way; she acknowledged the different contribution made by the mentor according to the individual, and acceded that their lesser skills would probably not always be so, saying:

> I've got a more in-depth knowledge of the whole course, whereas the mentor may have a more superficial idea of roughly what's in each module, and an in-depth knowledge of the student's competence and learning requirements for the particular module they are mentoring. There are particular things such as giving feedback to students. Because I've done a teaching course I've had experience in being able to give critical feedback in a supportive way. Some of them who've been in a more managerial position might have got those skills, but mentors at staff nurse level have probably never been in a position where they've had to give feedback to people before. [Also], I have more skills and knowledge of reflection at the moment, [but] I would hope that mentors would reach that level with more experience in mentoring.

All described their actual roles as being different, with the main two areas being that of the 'every-day' working with the students and the assessment of students. Felicity talked about the mentor as being the main 'reference point' for the student in the clinical placement, and Beth and Ann considered it 'to be the role of the mentor, and not the lecturer practitioner, to work alongside the students'. Similarly, Ellen 'relied very much on mentors doing most of the day-to-day discussion, carrying the students through, facing up to very difficult issues'.

In relation to the validation of the learning contract, Felicity's description of the differences in roles was consistent with the views of the others.

> The mentor works alongside the student, gives them immediate feedback on what they are doing and helps them to reflect and validates what the student did. The student self-assesses, but the mentor validates that the student was there when she said she was, and that either she performed better than her self-assessment or she had ideas of grandeur and needed to consider this and that. The lecturer practitioner then assesses the reflection.

Beth identified a problem about the perception of mentors as being the assessors of students. As she said:

> This is an issue that has got a bit fudged over the last year or 18 months. Some mentors think they are there to say the students are good, bad or indifferent. But they are there to *validate* what went on because they have been alongside them. It's my job to assess the quality of the work which has been validated by the mentor. I ask the mentor at the end what they think the grade of this work is, but that's not because I'm dependent on them. My assessment is the one, though I think it's important they see how grades are determined.

When comparing their roles with those of lecturers, two main, though linked, differences were suggested. First, all argued that they had a much greater contextual awareness and recent clinical knowledge that they could draw on. For example, Felicity talked about 'being in touch' and said:

> I know what's going on in the real world. I know what's possible. For example, how to help the student to prioritize, and to cut corners safely, still adhere to principles but use a quicker way of doing things to get the same result. Lecturers are basing what they think is achievable on their past experience which may be out of date and is clouded with time.

Second, all agreed that practice was complex, and suggested that because they were 'immersed in the practice setting', they were far more able to understand the complexities than lecturers 'who never set foot in practice'. They were then able to relate this better to the students. Beth and Ann in particular linked this to their actual physical presence on the ward. For example, Ann said:

> Because I am there, I know what is going on in the ward – the kinds of things that students here meet on a day-to-day basis. The lecturers don't have that advantage.

And when talking to a visitor Beth explained:

> One of the things about having teaching in a practice setting is that practice is very complex. Tutors are divorced from context. If I am there I can *see* the context, and exactly what they are involved in – students are unhappy about being criticized when their tutors don't know the context.

Implicit in Beth's remarks was also the idea that students should be judged on their clinical performance only by those who know the setting well, and that it was easier for the lecturer practitioner to challenge the student in these circumstances. Indeed, Beth contrasted her current role with her previous experience as a tutor, saying:

> I've failed students before [as a tutor] and you've been slightly working with your hand behind your back, fingers crossed, hoping that they'll swallow the line of argument you're presenting, 'cos you haven't actually been there with them.

Other aspects of difference that were raised included the lecturer practitioners' responsibility for module planning in relation to practice modules, with Felicity suggesting that 'most of the time the lecturer practitioners felt they knew best as far as the practice modules were concerned'. Conversely, although some lecturer practitioners were involved in the planning of theoretical modules – including all four studied – this was considered a minor and relatively unusual aspect of their roles compared with the lecturers, who had a major responsibility in this respect.

Conclusions regarding the role in relation to student learning

Charlotte and David had left before students were present in their clinical areas in practice modules, and thus their involvement in student learning within the undergraduate programme was limited to module planning.

Ann described her role in relation to student learning as having four main parts, in addition to module planning: 'providing the right clinical learning environment which was the early development work and the work [she] continued to do on the ward to maintain those standards; student supervision ... and guidance; marking their contract with the mentor; and preparing mentors ...'.

Similarly, Beth's role had four interlinked and related parts that contributed towards student learning as well as the module planning.

First she was there 'to manage the environment in which students are placed'. But, as she said, the ramifications of this extended beyond the students:

> It's quite clear in the job description that you're responsible for the clinical learning environment. It's the whole environment, so that everyone is pursuing the same beliefs about educating in practice ... Students are part of that, but they are not the only people who can reap the benefits of that environment.

Second, she argued that she 'facilitated learning by working through mentors', third, by direct contact with students, and fourth, by the assessment process.

Felicity was less engaged in developing the clinical environment, but otherwise her role was similar to Ann and Beth's. In addition, she had herself been a mentor. The emphasis in Ellen's role appeared to be much more on the two aspects of working through mentors and assessment, though she, too, had some direct contact with students, she had been a mentor and co-mentor, and she was involved in planning modules.

In conclusion, there were a number of key aspects that emerged. First, the views they held about, and the actions they took to achieve student learning appeared to be broader than traditional notions of facilitating learning as exemplified in the past by nurse tutors or ward staff. Conversely, all spent little or no time in some of the pursuits considered to be characteristic of nurse educators, such as traditional clinical teaching and lecturing. This seemed both because they did not see them as part of or appropriate to the role, and because of the limited time available.

Second, though there was a definite pattern in relation to some of the activities – notably assessment and module planning – the way they went about their jobs and the strategies they employed varied. So, for example, whereas Ann and Beth talked about managing the clinical learning environment in its totality, Ellen and Felicity focused more on supporting mentors and working through them. And whilst Ellen and Felicity considered that occasionally it was appropriate to be the mentor for students, the other two never did.

Third, on the whole there were few problems that the lecturer practitioners attached to this part of their jobs, except that they were having to develop the work as they went along since many of the activities were new – such as module planning, assessment by learning contract, and facilitating learning through reflection on practice – and there was a sense of 'having to work out a great deal for themselves'. Further, they were concerned about the future when the student numbers would have greatly increased, and the effect this would have on their workload.

And fourth, all articulated differences especially between their roles and those of mentors and lecturers. In relation to mentors, there seemed to be two considerations – that mentors would always be the people to work most closely clinically with the students, but also that the role of the mentors would be likely to change in the future as they 'became more skilled and knowledgeable', both about the programme and about facilitating student learning.

The education element of the role for the survey LPs

From the in-depth study, a distinction emerged between those activities that were seen to be facilitating student learning, such as curriculum development, and mentor preparation and support, and those where there was direct student contact or involvement, such as teaching or assessment. All the activities that the six LPs had engaged in were presented as possible components of the educational aspect of the lecturer practitioner role in the survey, and respondents were asked to indicate on a scale the amount of time spent on the activity – a great deal of time, quite a lot of time, some time, very little time, or no time at all. (The percentages indicate the proportion of the 55 respondents replying in this way.) Table 1 shows the results for those

Table 1 Time spent by survey LPs on activities in support of student learning

	Great deal of time	Quite a lot of time	Some time	Very little time	No time
Being member of module team	15% (F)	49% (B, E)	29%	5%	0%*
Being module or course leader	24% (E, F)	38% (B)	13%	4%	20%*
Supporting mentors in clinical area	5% (B)	55% (E, F)	27%	7%	5%
Curriculum development	18% (E, F)	25% (B)	35%	16%	4%*
Preparing mentors	5%	36% (B, E, F)	51%	5%	2%
Attending other meetings	1% (B)	20% (E, F)	49%	24%	5%*
Attending 'Poly' meetings	2%	10% (F)	53% (B, E)	27%	7%

* Figures do not add up to 100% because of missing data for one respondent.
(B) Beth, (E) Ellen, (F) Felicity.
$N = 55$.

aspects that were in support of student learning and Table 2, aspects where there was actual student contact. By way of comparison, the responses of Beth (B), Ellen (E) and Felicity (F) are indicated on the tables.

In terms of the proportions of respondents indicating that they spent either a great deal or quite a lot of time on an activity, by far the most time-consuming activity for the lecturer practitioners as a whole was assessing students. This matched the findings of the in-depth study. Linked with this was the moderation of learning contracts and student assignments, and 62% of lecturer practitioners in the survey spent a great deal or quite a lot of time on this. Similar percentages – 64% and 62% of survey lecturer practitioners – pertained for being a member of the module team and module leadership respectively, though in the case of the latter, 20% had no involvement at all with being a module leader. Conversely, it appears to have been a deliberate strategy, with many of the lecturer practitioners to restrict their attendance at meetings and only 12%

Table 2 Time spent by survey LPs on activities involving student contact

	Great deal of time	Quite a lot of time	Some time	Very little time	No time
Assessing students	18% (E, F)	56% (B)	20%	2%	2%*
Moderation	20% (B, E, F)	42%	31%	5%	0%*
Leading seminars	9%	45% (B)	42% (E)	2% (F)	0%*
Having student tutorials	11%	42% (B, E)	35% (F)	11%	0%*
Having sessions on reflection with students	15%	31% (B)	38% (E, F)	11%	5%*
Being a personal tutor to students	5%	29% (E, F)	36% (B)	16%	9%**
Giving lectures	4%	24%	40% (B)	22% (E, F)	9%*
Working with students in the clinical area	5%	16%	27% (B, F)	33% (E)	15%*
Being a mentor	7%	9%	31% (F)	16%	33% (B, E)**
Running support groups for students	0%	9% (E)	22%	24%	42% (B, F)**

* Figures do not add up to 100% because of missing data for one respondent.
** Figures do not add up to 100% because of missing data for two respondents.
(B) Beth, (E) Ellen, (F) Felicity.
$N = 55$.

claimed to spend significant amounts of time in this way. This finding concurred with the experience of Beth and Ellen, but not Felicity, who suggested she spent 'quite a lot of time' in such meetings. None the less, the same three LPs spent 'quite a lot of time' in special group meetings, such as Assessment of Practice Group and the Lecturer Practitioner Forum, whereas only 21% of survey lecturer practitioners spent either a great deal or quite a lot of time on the activity.

It is interesting to consider the four least time-consuming student-related activities. It was evident that the six LPs spent very little or (for Felicity) only some time on giving lectures. This compared with over a quarter (28%) of the survey lecturer practitioners who spent a great deal or quite a lot of time, 40% who spent some time and just under a third who spent little or no time. On balance, therefore, giving lectures tended to be engaged in somewhat more by survey lecturer practitioners than by the six LPs. Even so, it still featured well down the list in terms of time allocated, suggesting that the term 'lecturer' practitioner was somewhat of a misnomer for many.

Working with students in the clinical area was another intriguing aspect in that the in-depth study had revealed that the four LPs spent very little time in this way. This appeared to match more closely with the survey lecturer practitioners in that 45% claimed to spend little or no time and nearly a third (30%) spent 'some time' working with students in the clinical area. Similarly, at the time of the survey, Beth and Ellen said that they spent no time as mentors themselves – compared with a third of all survey lecturer practitioners – and Felicity spent 'some time' as a mentor – again compared with just over a third of survey lecturer practitioners (34%).

Whilst Ellen had run support groups for students, this was not so for the other three LPs. Likewise 42% of survey lecturer practitioners did not run student support groups at all, and only 9% spent any significant amount of time doing so.

In terms of their feelings about the educational aspect, in the questionnaire Beth was quite satisfied, but Ellen and Felicity wanted to change aspects, e.g. spend less time in departmental meetings and more time working alongside students. It seems that survey lecturer practitioners were slightly happier than the four LPs in that 50% were 'very satisfied' or 'quite satisfied', although almost a third (31%) would like to spend more time on such aspects as working clinically with students (several mentions), mentor support and preparation (several mentions), preparing seminars, reading and curriculum development. Six (11%) would like to spend less time on meetings (several mentions), moderation and administration. Four survey lecturer practitioners were not at all satisfied with the educational aspects of their role and they raised some interesting issues such as the 'unfair distribution of education work in the Department, low standards of some staff, the lack of involvement of some in course development' and the consequent burden on others; the 'terrific pressure of time' and the 'unfair student/LP ratios'. One felt that the enormous number of competing (educational) demands resulted in her 'not doing anything very well'.

The views of others about the LP's role in student learning

Finally, mentors and team leaders, students and educators had perspectives to offer about the part they felt their lecturer practitioners – Ann, Beth, Ellen and Felicity – played in student learning.

Mentors' and team leaders' views

All of the group agreed that the role of the lecturer practitioner in relation to student learning started with the planning, implementation and evaluation of the modules and included 'the overall responsibility for the students in clinical areas'. Further, there was agreement that the lecturer practitioner was 'jointly responsible' with the mentor for the assessment of the students, but that the lecturer practitioners 'had the final say' within the moderation procedures.

The group quite overtly compared their own role in this process with that of the lecturer practitioner, and herein lay insights into how it operated in practice. The lecturer practitioners were felt to be 'much more involved overall with the course and especially the modules', and the mentors were there on the ward, 'providing the clinical nursing', the 'day-to-day supervision and guidance', 'nurturing the students to become responsible and competent practitioners' and generally working much more closely with the students. Two made the distinction between practical and theoretical activities, some talked about mentors and lecturer practitioners working at different levels, and several talked about 'specific nursing things' and 'more general aspects'. For example,

> Mine [as a mentor] is more like a practical role to do with the clinical side of nursing. Beth is there more on the theoretical side – marking and bringing in research, that sort of thing. She is there for guidance and support, but at a high level.

> I am there to teach and demonstrate the practicalities of nursing care. Anything they want to discuss on a larger issue, or a more

general point, they go to Ellen about; for example, on ethics or their own personal coping.

'Working at a different level' seemed to be linked with the programme, and with expectations and standards. For example, 'Felicity is more at the level of the course; she knows far more about that than we do and what is expected of the students during the module'. And, 'Ellen knows the overall standard that students should be at.'

Three described a difference between the kind of teaching they engaged in. For example, one contrasted her 'clinical teaching' to that of the lecturer practitioner who was much more involved in 'lecturing' and 'running seminars'. Another said:

I don't actually teach them in the same way as the lecturer practitioner; I'm there more to facilitate the learning, by being a role model, by working alongside the student, by offering support.

And a third said: 'as a mentor you teach, but it's more clinical rather than theoretical', with again the implication being that the lecturer practitioner role was related more to aspects of theory.

Several made a distinction between their role and that of the lecturer practitioner in relation to problem-solving. Typically, as one mentor said:

I am there for the day-to-day things about the ward and the nursing. The student would come to me in the first instance if she had problems, but say it was about the course, or what the module was about – perhaps something I couldn't help with – or that they weren't getting on with their learning contract, or maybe that they didn't like me, then they would go to the lecturer practitioner.

In respect of assessment, and the learning contract, three mentioned that students were aware of the assessment role of the lecturer practitioner. As one said: 'They find me more approachable because they know that at the end of the day it's Felicity who decides on their final grade.' And 'I was there to help them rather than to quiz them, and be strict with them. Beth was there to have the final say, and they knew that.'

Three talked about the differences between the ongoing assessment, which they saw as the role of the mentor, and the marking of the learning contract and the giving of the final grade, which they saw as the responsibility of the lecturer practitioner. For example:

I was responsible for the assessment on the ward, very much so, because Felicity wasn't there working with them. She left it up to us to assess them, to use our own skills of observation and

> experience to judge what they were up to. She assessed their written work [in the learning contract] but because I was the one who had worked with them I could say, I don't think what she's written tallies with what she actually did, how she comes across.
>
> Although the overall assessment through the learning contract was a joint responsibility between me and Ann, on a day-to-day basis it was down to me.

All considered that in practice the marking of the learning contract was a joint activity, or almost always so. In terms of what actually happened, often the student was asked to self-assess, followed by the mentor saying what she felt. Mentors expected the lecturer practitioner to advise on the grading criteria, and almost half suggested that the actual final decision on grading was that of the lecturer practitioner. But one was only happy about this when her views concurred with those of the lecturer practitioner, since she argued: 'I felt that as I had worked with the student all the time I knew much more about her than the lecturer practitioner.' Nevertheless, she did concede that 'officially' the lecturer practitioner had the responsibility for grading, and that she as the mentor was not as familiar with the course and therefore the expectations of the students.

Two mentioned the problem that they had sometimes experienced in this process – of a difference between the student in practice and what they wrote in the learning contract. Here they considered their role was paramount to advise the lecturer practitioner and inform the consequent grade, yet they acknowledged that the lecturer practitioner could stand back and see things differently because she had not been involved. Thus:

> Something I found very difficult with [the student] was that clinically her practice was excellent and I was certainly quite happy to give her an 'A' for her practice. Separately the learning contract was excellent, her depth of insight was very good. But I was finding it very difficult to tie the two together. This was something I had to keep picking her up on towards the end of her placement. I was trying to say very gently that I wasn't seeing any evidence of what it was she was achieving on the ward in her learning contract. That was the one thing that was holding me back from saying I was going to give her an A, and I advised on a B+. But when the lecturer practitioner and I looked at the contract together, the lecturer practitioner could see the connections and pointed them out. So I was reassured.

A minority spontaneously saw an important aspect of the role of the lecturer practitioner in ensuring student learning (sometimes the *most* important facet) as 'working through the mentors to achieve good learning for students'. This was done by 'mentor preparation', 'the general professional development of mentors' and by 'the support of mentors in the clinical setting'. One team leader suggested that the main role of the lecturer practitioner in relation to student learning was 'certainly not to be a mentor herself, but rather to get the learning environment right'. This she did through 'every aspect of her role – clinical, managerial, education, research, and so on'.

Many of the mentors and team leaders had a much more hazy knowledge of what their lecturer practitioner did when she was off the ward. Several said that they assumed she must spend 'a fair bit of time lecturing in the Poly', a suggestion that was far from the truth with these particular four LPs, as indicated above.

Students' perspectives

In relation to the views of students on the lecturer practitioner's role in their learning, there was a tendency for all the students explicitly or implicitly to compare the role of lecturer practitioner with that of the mentor. There was some commonality in the ways they described this, and considerable agreement with the views of the mentors as expressed above. In the main, the lecturer practitioner was seen as the 'co-ordinator' with a role that is broader and related to the whole module, rather than providing the 'close guidance on everyday work' given by the mentor. Also, the lecturer practitioner was thought to be 'more knowledgeable about the learning contracts' and the person 'who was ultimately responsible for the assessment', although the mentor 'does have a role in validating performance' throughout the placement. Further, the lecturer practitioner was expected to give 'more academic input', both in general in relation to the programme and in providing suggestions for reading. The problem-solving capacity of the lecturer practitioner was recognized in the following typical comments:

> If anything on the ward was wrong, in the first instance I would always go to my mentor. If it was a broader thing, say something to do with the module, or if I had a problem with my mentor, I would go to [the lecturer practitioner].

> The lecturer practitioner's role in relation to her particular bunch of students is to keep an eye on where they're going, keep them on the right course and be available if there are any problems, but not to have direct involvement with them.

Conversely, one student did see the role of the lecturer practitioner quite differently, but this appeared to be closely related to the particular student and to the nature of the relationship deliberately formed with the lecturer practitioner. Thus:

> Ann was the first lecturer practitioner who actually practised with me on the ward, and I saw her practising, so she ... led by example. She actively provided plenty of opportunities for me to work with her both on and off the ward.

Apart from these activities and the ones that are described in the section on the nature of the role, such as the seminars and support groups, there was an impression gained from several of the students that the lecturer practitioners were not felt to be particularly important in their clinical learning on the ward, even if they valued them in other ways. For example:

> My mentor was really the main person; I only went to see my lecturer practitioner if I had problems or to discuss my learning contract.

> Whilst I was on the ward the contact was really with the mentor. But I knew I could always go to the lecturer practitioner if I needed other help, even though she always seemed to be very busy.

> I learnt from the whole team. I did see Ann from time to time working on the ward and that was helpful, but obviously her job is not there to work alongside us; that's more for the team.

The views did seem to vary, however, according to the circumstances of the lecturer practitioner. For example, there was a tendency for those students working on Ann, Beth and Felicity's own wards to mention seeing them on the ward, whereas students on placement on the other wards in Ann and Beth's units, and in Ellen's unit, tended to see them only in seminars, group meetings, during the marking of the learning contract and when a special visit or meeting had been arranged.

The views of educators

The educators appeared to see a great deal of similarity between their own role as 'facilitators of student learning' and that of the lecturer practitioner, except that the focus of the latter was different – being based in clinical settings – as was the amount of time they could spend on educational activities.

They tended to have a broader view than either the mentors or the students themselves, seeing the wider 'Poly' activities, the module development and mentor development as equally important in student learning as any direct contact they might have with the student. For example,

> I'd see a very skilled lecturer practitioner as working very much more through the mentors who in turn work with students. It is an indirect relationship in facilitating students by the preparation of mentors.

> The lecturer practitioner has to make sure that the mentors are well selected and are competent. That's vital to ensure student learning.

Both lecturers talked about the role of the lecturer practitioner in reflection. As one said: 'initially, at least until the mentors are able to do it, the lecturer practitioner should be facilitating the reflection of the students', and another, 'the lecturer practitioner helps in the process of critical reflection on practice'. One of the lecturers also stressed the importance of the lecturer practitioner as being 'ultimately accountable for the learning experience, and having the final decision about grading the module'.

Conclusion

Typically, the main part that lecturer practitioners in the in-depth study felt they played in student learning was that of facilitating the learning through others, especially the mentors; by the mechanisms of such aspects as assessment and the encouragement of reflection; via the enhancement of clinical areas where students were placed as effective learning environments; and indirectly through the curriculum development activities they were engaged in. This was mirrored within the survey and in the main confirmed by the views of others, except for an erroneous assumption on the part of many ward nurses that they 'lectured in the Poly' more than was the case.

Chapter 6

Theory and practice

Lecturer practitioners as a solution to problems of theory and practice in nursing has been a pervasive theme of other chapters – the rationale and plans for the lecturer practitioners, and the context in which LP posts have been established. In this respect, three questions were posed which the research attempted to answer: how are lecturer practitioners conceiving issues of theory and practice? how in reality are they dealing with such issues? and are there problems related to this? This chapter explores first what was found in the in-depth study, then in the survey, and finally from the study of the different perspectives.

The six LPs and issues of theory and practice

There was no mention at all of issues to do with theory and practice in the early stage of the in-depth study with one exception. Ellen, when reviewing her role, suggested that she was 'conscious of truly linking theory and practice and generating the progression of nursing and nurses through all aspects of [her] role'. However, it was not evident at this point how she felt she was achieving the link.

In the final stage, there was a tendency for them to talk about theory and practice mainly in two ways – first, in respect of students and student learning, and second, by giving a wider view of theory and practice.

Theory and practice and student learning

All four seemed to believe that they should either enable students to, or ensure that students did, apply theory to practice, where theory meant both knowledge gained from literature and knowledge derived from the other – theoretical – modules, and practice meant what they actually did in the clinical setting, and described in the learning contract. This, for the lecturer practitioners, was very much 'part of the students' learning process'. For example, Ann talked about 'being impressed when students weave in theory to their practice'. When asked about this she said:

> They can do it in two ways. They can either read and say 'I'd really like to try that out in practice', and then tell me how they are trying it, whether it worked or not. Or they can do something and when they recount it to me, I say, well Watson [a nurse theorist] has talked about that, why don't you look at what she writes about 'hope'. And then quite often they'll say, after they've read it, 'it seems my experience does concur with Watson'.

She also referred to encouraging the student to 'blend theory with practice' and when asked, in interview, how she got students to do this, she said:

> I specifically ask them questions, perhaps in a tutorial, to get them to do this. I invite the student to tell a story – for example, about a patient who wouldn't do what she [the student] wanted him to do. The student said she was in a dilemma. She felt she had no authority and she also knew the philosophy of the ward which is for people to have information and control and make decisions for themselves. So we started talking about the interpersonal skills module, because I knew they'd done negotiation that week, to see if she could come up with any useful tactics. In that way, I was getting her to think about what she had learnt from a theoretical module.

Similarly, Beth described how, when talking to students in the seminar or whilst they were on the ward, she posed different perspectives or points of view (in other words, 'different theoretical positions') and thus 'enriched their understanding'. This, she argued, was one of the ways she enabled students to draw on theory.

Ellen specifically mentioned how she was conscious during module planning of the relationship between this and theoretical ideas that would be useful for the students. She explained:

> When I'm planning my module, I'm aware of such things as theories of caring. Then when I'm, say, presenting the weekly lecture – or especially in discussion in the support group – I'll throw some ideas at the students about these theories.

Felicity said that when she was with students she was often 'aware of the relationship between the theoretical inputs and practice'. She did not say what action, if any, she took, but she identified a problem that 'a lot of the students were not seeing the relevance of their theory modules to their practice'. This she sought to address by having discussions with students 'to try and draw those things together'.

Further, she was observed talking with students about what they had seen and asked questions about how this equated to what they had done in other modules.

Specifically in relation to learning contracts, Felicity asked the students all the way through to support what they were saying with literature, and she made several references to the relationship between the students' practice and their knowledge of, for example, physiology, or the literature on particular areas of research such as preparation of children for admission to hospital. She remarked more than once, 'that is a good example where you have related practice to theory', and she expected the 'A grade' student to do this critically, saying:

> That's how I see them applying theory to practice and practice to theory, so they're not just accepting a theory as being right. They're looking at the context of the situation on the ward and thinking, is this going to fit on this particular ward.

Beth both asked the student to provide examples of her practice 'to illustrate the textbook view given' and, conversely, to 'provide evidence from the literature' to back up the points made in the contract. Ann attempted to get the student to draw on the 'theory' they had learnt from other modules. For example, during one validation she said to the student, 'you need to be pulling theory into your practice a lot more' and after the event, she said to the mentor that she thought the student should not get a higher mark because she was not analytical enough or relating her experience to theory. Indeed, throughout the process she made several comments about the need for students to provide evidence that they were drawing on theory to help understand and explain the practice.

Felicity was also 'conscious of relating theory and practice' in the group reports, another part of the assessment process, but contrasted the standard of this with the learning contracts. She explained:

> In group reports, quite a high percentage of marks are for application of theory to practice and implications for practice, and generally speaking that's quite poorly done. I think in learning contracts students are more acutely aware that they are trying to apply theory to practice and when it comes to group report they seem to forget that, because it's more of a theoretical exercise we're asking them to do. Or maybe they need more help to see the links. When they're working on the wards they can see the links because their mentors might be pointing them out, saying there's some literature about that situation you've seen, whereas when they're doing group report they've not got anyone there who can

make sense of what they might have seen, and apply it to the theory they might have read. So that's really where I come in.

There was also debate about whether the students were deriving theory from practice and the part played by the lecturer practitioner in this. Ann was cautious. In a workshop, another lecturer practitioner had said, 'the development of theory from practice – that's what this course is about', but Ann had replied she was not sure it was quite like that. When asked to expand, she referred to the short term, and to her longer-term aspirations saying:

> I think that's a bit pretentious. It's not what the *course* is about. But hopefully it'll be what the *Department* is about in ten years time. I hope that we will always hang on to this notion of practice being a fundamental source of knowledge for nursing and that we will look into reflection and learning from experience, and begin to do some good work in terms of generating nursing knowledge, but that's well in the future. I haven't seen a lot of theory generation from the practice of our students at the moment . . . However, I do feel I have a part to play in this – by doing it myself, through discussion with mentors and students.

Similarly, Felicity considered that 'we should be generating theory from practice', but that nursing was not at that stage yet in that there needed to be more time to research and evaluate. She felt that the nearest the students got was 'taking theories and modifying them to fit'. Conversely, Ellen considered that by the end of the third year of the course the students were beginning to 'develop their own theories'. She said:

> I see learning from reflection from action as the first stepping stone. If they can reflect in action, what they are really doing is devising their own theories on the hoof about what's going on.

In this respect she saw it as her role to assist in the process of students reflecting on practice.

Wider perspectives on theory and practice

In the third stage, it was evident that in addition to the importance they attached to aspects of theory and practice for students, all of them had a broader perspective, both in terms of their views of the issues and the part that they as lecturer practitioners could play. For example, when Felicity talked about theory and practice, she quite explicitly referred to two levels, a global level and the more specific level of the relationship to students. She explained the first as follows:

Theory and practice are to do with some of the key concepts or aspects that we value, like holistic care, continuity of care and parent partnership, and trying to develop things in practice that take on board those concepts. It's to do with generating a philosophy for practice based on all those ideas and then putting it into action.

She gave further examples of the wider notions or concepts that should be put into practice, such as 'nurse accountability, autonomy, self-care', and said the mechanism by which such approaches could be promoted was either through the 'use of nursing models', or by using 'standard setting' procedures. Felicity saw that she had a major role to play, first of all in the development of a ward philosophy which embodied the above mentioned principles, even though she might be working through others such as the staff nurses to achieve it. But she felt that although a great deal had already been achieved, 'they had still got a long way to go'.

She also made an important link between this and the other level of conceptualization, saying:

If we get those wider things right, theory and practice will automatically be matched for the students. When the [planning] group were talking about the learning contract I found it quite difficult initially to identify with that as the starting point of putting theory and practice together because I saw that at quite a low level and there were higher, wider things to be considered first.

In the second stage, whilst commenting on her own role, Beth made the distinction described above of developing theory *from* practice and using theory *in* practice in relation to herself. She 'reflected' upon one of the primary patients she had been nursing for several months, and how much she had learnt from that person, for example, about how a younger person copes with disability and 'what life was like in hospital for a patient'. In doing this, she concluded that 'maybe there is something in getting theory from practice by looking at cases like that [because] it's not exactly the way it's described in books currently'.

In the third stage, Beth, too, talked about 'the more global level' of theory and practice which was to do with where she got her 'new knowledge and new theory' from. She accepted that she learnt experientially, which both contributed to theory (as knowledge) as well as challenging it, though she was 'not entirely sure how'. She described how the experience of nursing particular patients 'raised issues for [her] that may or may not currently have a theoretical knowledge base, and that each experience may have to be treated on an individual basis'. But she was uncertain as to whether she had got any further than 'recognizing that challenges for knowledge come from a variety of places', since though she may draw on sociology or psychology it 'never tells you the whole story'.

She attributed this confusion in part to the complexity of nursing practice, and the novelty in nursing of having to say from where knowledge emanates:

> The way nursing's going now, you have to keep so many balls in the air when you're looking after a patient. It's not just physical care and reference to the life sciences for your information. It is quite a new area for nursing to actually clearly describe what knowledge is being used in a particular situation, and the fact that some knowledge is being adulterated a bit to fit this unique situation.

Ann, whilst not actually referring to another level of concept regarding theory and practice, saw her role as 'developing the practice of nursing, both herself and through the staff nurses', and she mentioned this when talking about the meaning of theory and practice. Ellen, too, talked about 'changing practice' and 'achieving a philosophy' as, in her mind, being the crux of the matter. She said:

> Maybe the essence of the lecturer practitioner's conception of theory and practice comes back to this authority to develop and change and identify where practice is going. That's really the issue and you are only then breaking it down to theory and practice. They are almost sidelines. You have got to ask the right questions, and you have to have your philosophy. At the end of the day, if we are talking about quality of nursing, we are talking about achieving our philosophy. You've got to be in there, looking forward and learning from looking backwards. That's where reflection comes in.

Lecturer practitioners as bridging a gap between theory and practice

All of them in some way addressed the issue of whether they considered there was a gap or disparity between theory and practice, and whether the lecturer practitioner had a role in this respect. Felicity considered that in part she was there to 'bridge the gap' for students, and gave two examples in particular – the application of knowledge between different modules and the utilization of research skills, saying:

One of the weaknesses of the course in general at the moment is that the students can't apply things between one module and another. That's coming out in third year students. They do modules on play and child psychology and they see the two things as totally separate. They can't see the links between the two without help.

With the research skills module, they can't see the point of that at all. I see it very much as my role to try to identify where students and nurses are using research skills. They're using the skills of observation and questioning in their daily work. A lot of the time people do use theory in practice – and vice versa – but they need to analyse their thinking. If they thought about it they would realize it's something they'd read or were aware of. But sometimes it's like Benner's intuition that isn't explicit.

Felicity added another dimension to the discussion when answering a question – posed by herself for a workshop of lecturer practitioners – about whether lecturer practitioners were the answer to the theory–practice question. She referred to the conditions necessary for this to be so, saying:

I think it is the perfect solution provided that the [clinical] patch for which you have responsibility and accountability is small enough to manage. I think that's one of the keys to why my workload is manageable, because I've only got one ward. But if you are going to have one lecturer practitioner over five wards they can't be anything more than clinical teacher and I don't then think they are a solution to the gap.

Ellen, too, saw it as 'one of the facets of the role' to 'bridge the gap', and felt that she was able 'to offer more in this respect than [she] did as a clinical teacher'. She gave two reasons, and again talked about the different levels:

I can do it at a more global level because I have the authority and can promote change in practice. One of the issues in terms of the lecturer practitioner role is to identify the gaps and to do something about them, for example, by setting up the research. On another level, with my module, the first two days were very much the theory introduction and I asked the students to give a very simple three positives and three negatives from the days for me to go away and think about. I then threw them back to the students and gave them the opposites from a practice point of view. In terms of bridging the gap in the module, the first point is to get over their attitude, their dilemmas in terms of cancer.

Beth, also, talked about the integration of theory and practice, and in doing so introduced a different, organizational dimension. She talked about the role as 'not being a personal bridge between theory and practice, but rather structural'. She continued that 'the structure is there and it stands to reason that theory and practice are brought more together', though she did not expand further on what she meant by this.

When thinking about whether she as a lecturer practitioner was a bridge between theory and practice, Beth said that 'at a very simplistic level' she was, this being illustrated by discussions between students and lecturer practitioners whereby questions are 'being posed backwards and forwards' and 'reference is being made to the literature'. However, at the wider level she was unsure whether lecturer practitioners were 'yet the bridge', since nursing knowledge, theory and practice were complex, the generation of new understanding about them was difficult and the relationship between them was elusive.

Conversely, Ann considered that it was inappropriate to talk about a theory–practice gap any more. Rather, for her, bringing theory and practice together in nursing meant 'talking about what happens in terms of experience, and what helps us to make experience more meaningful'. She suggested this could be done in various ways, for example:

> You can read the theory first and apply it to practice, but then you've got to reflect upon whether it worked or not and why it worked or not, and what was going on at the time etc. Or you can do it the other way round, saying this happened to me in practice, is there anything that could help me to understand it better, anything written?

She related the learning opportunity this provided to her own experience, saying:

> When I've read something that confirms my practice it makes me feel better about my practice, more confident about it, and I really begin to develop my practice at a much faster rate than I did before. This is what I'm hoping for the students.

Outstanding concerns related to theory and practice

In terms of outstanding problems in relation to theory and practice, Felicity and Beth were the only two who talked at any length about these. Felicity identified two. As indicated before, she recognized that there was still some way to go putting into practice the best philosophy of paediatric care, and she outlined a contextual problem about the organization of the course itself which militated against the effective integration of theory and practice. First, there was an issue about students being involved in concurrent modules which meant that they 'could not get a sufficient run at practice':

> There are some problems with the modular course and the way that practice is organized. We are expanding continuity of care as important, yet sometimes the students have difficulty getting continuity of practice in order to begin to see that happening. They are doing four different modules, and juggling their timetable; you try and suggest that they might do a block of four/five days on the ward to get into the swing of it, but they find that's not possible because they've got other modules in the way.

Second, the opportunity to have a period of theory followed immediately by consolidation in practice was missing. As she said:

> There was some value in having a block introduction to all the key things they were going to meet in the particular learning experience, then to have that experience, and then to consolidate what they'd learnt and bring it all back. But that doesn't happen with a modular course. They might have something about principles of child care and the child with fluid electrolyte problems, i.e. a neonate with a colostomy, and it could be some months or even the following year before they even meet one. I think that's always been a problem, but I think its been compounded by the modular course.

Felicity felt that a partial solution to this was to concentrate more on the principles of care, for example, the theory of the child with fluid electrolyte problems, and then spend more time applying those principles to whatever they happened to see in the ward areas, rather than even mentioning patient conditions at all.

Beth felt that it was early days in the development of the lecturer practitioner role and that the potential had yet to be realized. She said:

> Potentially, lecturer practitioners with good support and resources could be quite significant in raising issues to be seriously explored and examined, and as a consequence of that you may see theory practice as one long word, without the 'and' in between. The issues have been identified by someone [whose role embodies theory and practice] and therefore the issues are not just looked at from a theory or practice point of view.

She also suggested that the Assessment of Practice Group was a forum where the practicalities of theory and practice were dealt with, in that whilst 'some of the issues tackled may seem superficially to be very clearly focused on a practical problem, they are possibly the symptom of an underlying change or development of how theory and practice are viewed'.

Conclusions regarding theory and practice issues

Since theory and practice issues were barely raised, if at all, in the first stage, there are no conclusions to draw about Charlotte's and David's understanding of their meaning and importance, nor any notion of what they did in practice.

It appears that Ann's conceptualization of theory–practice issues was not so much of there being a disparity between the theory that students learnt and the actual practice of nursing, but rather that (theoretical) knowledge is there either to be drawn on to guide practice or to help understand practice. And in terms of what Ann actually did, and the strategies she employed, these comprised asking students direct questions to either get them to think about theoretical knowledge, or to test out their theoretical knowledge, referring students to sources of nursing knowledge in the hope that students would use them, and having as one of her criteria for marking students' contracts the extent to which students have related theory and practice.

Beth had a general as well as a specific concept of theory–practice. The former was to do with the nature of knowledge for nursing – a 'theory of practice'. However, she felt that lecturer practitioners were both in their infancy in relation to understanding the wealth of knowledge (theory) that informed practice and, further, were not all likely to take the kind of intellectual approach necessary for achieving this understanding. And whilst she did use strategies with students to try to get them to consider different theoretical perspectives on practice, this was related to what was already known, and did not expand the boundaries of new knowledge.

Ellen had difficulty conceptualizing them as two totally separate things 'as [she] saw the role as so unified and . . . didn't think about theory on the one hand and practice on the other'. As she said: 'I hardly ever stop and think about the difference, because the whole point is you're pulling them together', and it did make sense to her to think of her role as attempting to bridge a gap between the two.

Felicity appeared to make two major types of distinction in relation to issues of theory and practice. The first was the process of relating theory to practice as compared with generating theory from practice. The second was the distinction between two levels of attention – global and more specific, the premise being that the two are interlinked in that if 'making a philosophy of nursing happen in practice' is achieved then there will be no issue about a disparity between theory and practice for students.

In conclusion, it appears that the major problems or issues of the theory–practice relationship which they considered their role should address were: to help students apply or use theory (gained from other modules and from the literature) in their practice, as well as to 'theorize' about their practice; and to develop, or assist in the development of, their clinical areas 'so that the practice better reflected theoretical notions about the nature of good nursing'. In these respects, they distinguished between two levels of theory/ practice – one related to the students and the other to do with the broader aims of the development of clinical practice.

The strategies they used to tackle the issues included: developing a philosophy within the clinical area 'so that theory would be realized in practice'; ensuring, for example, through their questioning that students were making connections between theory and practice; being a source of both theoretical and practice knowledge for students; and encouraging students to reflect on and to theorize about their practice, mainly in the learning contracts, but also in group and individual discussions. All but one thought that it was appropriate to talk about a disparity or gap between theory and practice, that they had a role in bridging that gap, and that although there was 'some way to go' they had been moderately successful in doing so already. One claimed that the existence of the role itself, as part of the 'new structure' for nursing and nurse education, was in itself a solution to the theory–practice problem, though this idea was not expanded and remained elusive.

They articulated outstanding concerns, the main ones being the development of their own practice and theories as new knowledge, and the development of students' ability to generate theory from their practice. Problems were also identified which were to do with the structure of the programme: the modular nature militated against the integration of knowledge between modules and the juxtaposition of the theoretical and practice modules.

The findings of the survey

The major issues or problems of the theory–practice relationship which the four LPs considered their role should address were put to the survey LPs. (The figures in brackets are the proportions of survey lecturer practitioners who agreed with these statements; they were able to indicate more than one possibility.) Thus tackling issues of theory and practice meant:

- ensuring the development of theory from practice and the application of theory to practice (78%);
- clarifying the nature of knowledge that informs professional nursing (67%);
- the two levels – the global level and the more specific level of matching theory and practice for students (62%);
- overcoming the disparity between what is taught in theoretical modules and the practice of nursing (60%).

The ways in which the four LPs tried to achieve this were suggested to the survey LPs – again the figures in brackets show the proportions of survey lecturer practitioners who agreed with these statements. Thus theory–practice issues were addressed:

- by encouraging students to reflect on their practice (98%);
- by ensuring (e.g. through their questioning) that students were making the connections between theory and practice (91%);
- by being a source of theoretical and practice knowledge for students (91%);
- by helping students to theorize about their practice (78%);
- by developing a philosophy for the clinical area so theory was realized in practice (65%).

As far as lecturer practitioners being the 'perfect solution to the theory–practice gap' was concerned, all but one of the four thought that it was appropriate to talk about a disparity or gap between theory and practice, that they had a role in bridging that gap, and that although there was 'some way to go' they had been moderately successful in doing so already. This was matched by 64% of LPs who thought they achieved it some of the time, 16% most of the time and 11% who did not achieve it at the moment but felt they would in the future. (The remainder – 9% – gave a range of sometimes quite complex 'other' answers to the question.)

The views of others

Mentors and team leaders, students, educators and managers all had views about issues of theory and practice.

Mentors' and team leaders' perspectives

Respondents were asked the questions: 'Lecturer practitioners are supposed to be bridging the theory–practice gap in nursing. Do you think they do this, and in particular your lecturer practitioner? If so how? If not, what are the problems?' Three said that they felt their lecturer practitioner did 'bridge the theory–practice gap' (in respect of Ann, Beth and Felicity), and one that she did not (in respect of Beth). The three explained how this was achieved as follows:

> Ann brought the theories she knew into practice on a day-to-day basis. She would encourage you to discuss certain aspects of patient care without pontificating about a certain person's theory, by encouraging you along a certain train of thought, and then she'd say 'I think you ought to read such and such'. She was constantly stimulating discussion and thought. Because she had the theoretical knowledge, she was able to discuss it from a knowledgeable point of view.

> She does it better than anywhere else I've ever worked. It's not perfect, but it's the best I've ever worked with. She's in touch, she's a familiar face to us, to the students. She's supportive to us, to the students. She brings theory on to ward because she allows staff nurses to develop the ward. She's developing our environment for us and we're helping her do it. Felicity has a lot of ideas, she understands the tensions, the stresses, the problems we have, because she's around. For the students, especially, she's brilliant because she's always around on the ward; she knows what they have to aim for because she's got the Poly basis.

> Beth [bridges the gap] because she knows her stuff and that comes across. She does this not only with the students, but also the staff. Therefore, you're getting the students thinking along those lines so they can see how it all relates together. Also, we all worked on the ward in very similar ways and Beth picked her staff – we were all very similar and put the same things across.

A further team leader talked about lecturer practitioners in general, but again agreed that they probably do bridge the gap, in the following ways:

> Since they have so many clinical days they are keeping in with clinical practice and hands-on care – I would imagine what they are teaching in the classroom is much more pertinent. They also do it by keeping themselves up-to-date, by having the clinical experience, taking a patient workload, working on the wards.

Conversely, one mentor suggested that her lecturer practitioner only partially bridged the gap 'because she does not have very much input on the ward . . . and because of the other commitments she's got'. She explained that the lecturer practitioner's main contact with the student was via the learning contract, and whilst the lecturer practitioner discussed what the student did in practice, primarily the contact was 'more theoretical'. One team leader suggested that the gap was not being bridged, but that the situation was far more complex than is first apparent.

> The potential is there but the theory and practice gap is not effectively bridged by having lecturer practitioners, because it's partly down to personality and the amount of theory that someone has got, has understood, and has internalized. Also, the extent to which they have made it meaningful in their practice, and the extent to which they communicate it to others. With tools such as reflection and learning contracts, there's more chance than in my training. But there is so much theory, and practice is so complex and varied that in some ways it's a futile task. So all you can do is try to promote an environment where neither one nor the other are mutually exclusive nor seen as superior. If you can do that you're getting somewhere.

Of those who did not give a definitive answer either way, but who were basically positive, one construed the issue as being about the lecturer practitioner's influence in research-based practice, as well as being about students. As she explained:

> Beth has always been interested in the trained staff. She has made me feel motivated to do things; I see her as very much influencing my practice and my wanting to develop myself. But obviously she is there for the students as well. She does this through the learning contracts. The students are using reflection and when they are reflecting on their practice and looking into research as they are doing it, they are seeing a link between what they have done and what they should be doing. Beth has been very valuable in helping them see that.

Another talked entirely about the development of the ward as the way to bring theory and practice together. Thus she said:

> I don't know how she managed it, but Ann always knew which direction she wanted the ward to go in and she had vision. But she never came across as being a dictator. She would wangle it so you thought it was your own and the ward's idea. She would listen and take account and let you do what you wanted. For example, on my last ward we had a communication book; I suggested it and Ann said, 'you get the book and try it out'. The ward was always changing with new ideas. It made the ward because everyone felt they were part of it. To me that's what bringing theory to practice was all about – breaking down the hierarchy, making nurses think

for themselves. The way she went about introducing primary nursing was very subtle. She knew what she was heading for.

Similarly, two mentors working with Ellen saw the issue as very much the development of practice and the trained nurses mainly through teaching; the provision of support and advice on standard setting; and the bringing of 'psychological theory (such as how to motivate people and achieve change) to practice'. Also, it happened 'on a one-to-one basis, for example, where Ellen graded a learning contract done by one of the nurses, or gave feedback on a plan for caring for a very ill patient'.

Finally, one mentor did not seem to consider that the lecturer practitioner herself bridged the gap since she 'concentrates more on the theory side of things'. However, in her mind the integration was achieved through the lecturer practitioner's work with mentors. She explained:

> I think the way she manages to link the theory with the practice is through us a lot, and the way we feed back to her and the way she works alongside us with the students. The lecturer practitioners set up the objectives and competencies that the students have to achieve, and it's through us that we enable them to do that. There's a definite link there. A lot of the competencies are wishy washy and hard to work out practically. However, Felicity will try to give us an example of how to get the student to achieve it.

Students' perspectives

The five students who were in their third year all agreed that their lecturer practitioner did bridge the gap between theory and practice, whereas the other two, both second years, said that the lecturer practitioner 'probably did', but talked about lecturer practitioners in general rather than their lecturer practitioner. However, though the ways in which group members felt this was achieved did not appear contradictory, all laid the emphasis on slightly different aspects. These differences appeared to be random rather than, for example, relating to a specific lecturer practitioner. Thus, one said that Ann brought theory and practice together by 'encouraging her [i.e. the student] to relate what she was doing in other theory modules to her practice', whereas another felt Ann did it especially by 'introducing [her] to texts'.

A third student suggested that it was 'the way Beth questioned [her] practice, mainly through the learning contract, that tested what theory [she] knew and made [her] more aware of the relationship'.

Her colleague emphasized the importance of the seminars in this respect, saying, 'it was mainly through the seminars that Beth did it, by asking us to draw on our experience and give her extra examples'.

A further student gave several ways in which Ellen achieved the integration, including the following:

> She does it by being in touch with what's going on in clinical practice, by herself having done the Master's course, by being involved in planning the modules and what goes into them. She also guides you to sources of information, and draws on her own experiences as well which was really helpful. It happens mainly because she straddles two worlds, academic and practice, and has a real empathy for both.

With the other two students who felt that 'probably' lecturer practitioners bridged the gap, one suggested they did it 'by engendering an atmosphere in the ward whereby nursing staff are encouraged to relate theory and practice', and the other talked more generally about the teaching sessions – the introductory seminars for the Growing Child Module – and how these 'tied in very well with practice'.

Educators' perspectives

Both lecturers and the education manager had conceptions of theory and practice that were far more complex in some ways than in either of the previous two groups. In effect, they all either rejected the 'simplistic' idea of the lecturer practitioner role being about bridging a gap between theory and practice, or considered that it did not go far enough. Instead, they talked about the core issue as one of the development of practice, and the elicitation of knowledge about practice. As one said:

> We've all talked about the theory–practice gap, and all have experienced that as the difference between what you learn in the classroom and what you do in the ward. To me the LP role is much bigger than that. It's about having these highly refined skills in a practice setting that can be used to actually examine and develop practice, and develop the body of knowledge about nursing.

The other lecturer articulated a similar view, saying:

> I think the whole notion of a theory–practice gap is wrong. It stems from a fundamental misunderstanding about the nature of professional education. If you look at what professional education is about, you start from practice and *then* you look at theory. And

perhaps the LP can say 'what is the knowledge base behind this?' Then if you look at reflective practice, which we do in the programme, it is about practice which is generating the awareness of the need for theory. That is a very different consideration than in traditional nurse education.

The education manager, too, stressed the importance of starting from practice by indicating that

the understanding of nursing has to be generated in practice – you cannot 'theorize' nursing in the same way as say sociology or psychology. The whole rationale for the LP – in fact for the programme – is to enable the analysis of practice, with the potential for the generation of knowledge taking place within practice.

Only one of the three, a lecturer, described how she considered this was actually done by one of the lecturer practitioners in the study. She said:

I think Felicity both examines practice and develops a body of knowledge. She does this by promoting critical thinking about practice, she uses established theoretical frameworks to organize her presentations and her learning experiences, but she doesn't leave it there. She facilitates practitioners to think about their practice, to be more analytical, to challenge the norm. She also comes in from the other side by getting undergrads to question their practice.

The other lecturer addressed the issue of the development of theory from practice, but whilst she said she would like to think that lecturer practitioners did go some way towards this, in reality 'the minutiae of day-to-day concerns militate against this', and she could not think of any lecturer practitioner 'who freed themselves enough to have the time to do it'. This was something, however, that she saw as the potential of the role.

Service managers' perspectives

The way in which service managers talked about theory and practice varied, but on the whole it was non-specific and superficial. One of them said that lecturer practitioners did bridge the gap, but gave no explanation as to why or how, beyond the fact that the 'system of education [had] changed'. The second was a little more expansive, but considered that there were limitations as to how far the lecturer practitioner could do this. Nevertheless, she suggested that her lecturer practitioner had 'given the staff nurses theoretical knowledge which they could use in practice'.

A third senior manager was quite sceptical. She argued that whilst 'sometimes the lecturer practitioner can bring theory and practice together', there were severe restrictions to this. She related her comments to her lecturer practitioner, saying that

> because of the students which take up a lot of her time, there is a lack of continuity with the ward and with the trained staff – the people who are actually practising theory – and you cannot change things unless you are *there* to change them. Whether or not it works if you've got an LP combined with senior nurse – which I've got some reservations about anyway – I'm not sure.

Finally, the Director of Nursing Service argued that his three colleagues did bridge the gap, but they did it in different ways. These were, however, all related to developing practice. He explained as follows:

> On the one hand, Felicity had great difficulty in influencing practice, but by the use of many tactics, including working through other people such as the staff nurses, she achieved it very successfully. Ann and Beth had an easier time because they truly had accountability for practice, at least on their own wards. They influenced practice because of a whole range of things, such as through the staff they appointed, by being role models, by allowing staff nurses to develop and by creating the right environment on the ward.

Conclusion

All the parts of the research showed the question of theory and practice in nursing and nurse education to be an intricate one, which in much of the literature has been portrayed far too simplistically. Clearly, lecturer practitioners do see themselves as tackling the whole arena and they were able to articulate ways in which they did so. These were often reinforced by others working with them. However, as indicated, perhaps most strongly by the educators, the issues involved are sophisticated and there is still some way to go. Clearly, though, the lecturer practitioner role has considerable potential to move in the right direction.

Chapter 7

The viability of the job

The viability of the job has been a concern from the very beginning. Chapter 3 indicated it to be a consideration even at the planning stage, and it was an issue throughout all stages of the research. In addition, there was the factor of whether or not the role was in reality a unified one, or did it fall into the same trap as other roles which were rejected in its favour. This chapter explores whether the job was in fact possible, and the problems that have been experienced with it, from the perspectives of the six LPs, the survey LPs and others working with the lecturer practitioners. It also discusses the issues of unification, and the views about the different models of lecturer practitioner.

Problems and challenges of the job

The main common problems or challenges experienced by the six lecturer practitioners at the different stages were related to: the size of the job; the necessity to take on aspects that were or should normally be the role of others; the busy-ness of the clinical areas; the inability to do parts of the job through lack of time; the newness of the role and the lack of clarity about it; and the perceptions of, and pressures from, others.

First, there was a concern amongst the majority that the job was 'actually' or 'potentially' too large. There seemed to be two related issues – one of the overall workload (amount) and the other to do with the number of different aspects (breadth). In the first stage, these were felt to be problematic by Charlotte, Ellen and Felicity, though not in a general sense by Beth. By the second stage, all were more involved in 'Poly' work than hitherto and were more acutely aware of the potential problems of the job in relation to size. It was still an issue in the third stage.

Second, and related to the size of the job, was the need for all of them to undertake work that they felt should not be part of their role. For example, in the first stage, David and Ellen had to take on the

Senior Nurse role, and both considered that it meant they were 'not operating as a proper lecturer practitioner because of the need to also be the senior nurse manager'. In addition, David felt frustrated at the excessive amount of 'real nursing' he was doing (because of the shortage of staff and other people's expectations). Ann and Beth were also concerned that they were having to undertake secretarial and administrative work that was time-consuming, and could 'more cost effectively' be done by a secretary. This appeared to be much less of a problem during the following two stages.

Third, all of them worked in busy clinical areas. For Charlotte, Ellen and Felicity it appeared to be a fact rather than a problem as such, whereas David stated: 'it's a very busy unit and I think nobody realized it was going to be so busy and that's a problem for me', and in doing so implied that in planning to locate a lecturer practitioner there that factor had not been taken into account. Beth talked about the times that she had to nurse on the wards because of staff shortages and for Ann too it was quite a concern. She spent a great deal of her time working on the ward, and many of the shifts worked were 'very busy' – with the result that she was 'simply looking after patients and not actually teaching'. By the third stage, Ellen had distanced herself from ward work, and Felicity no longer felt responsible for ward staffing. Ann and Beth felt they had to relate their clinical work to periods of busy-ness, but that staffing was improved, and the staff were able to cope better on the ward in their absence.

Fourth, there were aspects of the job that, primarily through lack of time, they were unable to do. For example, in the early days four wanted to work more as primary nurses on a regular basis and none of them had engaged in research to any extent, despite this being part of their brief as they saw it. By the final stage, there were still aspects that either they wanted to engage in (e.g. research) or that they felt were expected of them, but that they were unable to achieve.

Fifth, the roles were new, both to the occupants and to the organization. There was a lack of clarity about them, and there were varying views and expectations of others as to the proper nature of the role. At first this was especially a worry for David and Felicity. Eventually this had largely been rectified for Felicity by discussion and negotiation, and by her being identified as the Service Delivery Unit (SDU) manager for the ward, a status she felt was obvious to others.

Finally, in the second stage, a new common problem had emerged. All felt the pressures upon them from 'the education and the service side' since the students were now in their wards and the lecturer practitioners' educational responsibilities had increased. This was evident, both in their need to 'fit other aspects around the students'

(Felicity and Ellen), and the feeling, most strongly expressed by Beth, of 'both sides [education and service] pushing to have more than 50%' of their time.

Strategies and conditions

Three main types of approach to make the job workable were apparent. First, there were those strategies that were within the control of the lecturer practitioners themselves such as – consistently working long hours, categorizing and planning the work, setting boundaries, assigning priorities, not doing parts of the job, and reconceptualizing the role. Second, there were strategies that were at least in part dependent on working with others such as – the development of others to take on aspects of the role, delegation, negotiating role boundaries with colleagues and clarifying the role. And third, there were certain conditions that were sought by the lecturer practitioners.

In terms of the strategies over which the lecturer practitioner did have control, initially, four out of the six consistently and deliberately worked longer hours than they were contracted for. It appears that working longer hours was considered both necessary and acceptable in order to 'get the job up and running'. Working long hours remained a feature of the next two stages also, although all found ways of ensuring that the hours worked reached a more manageable and acceptable level.

Second, at all stages they categorized and planned the work in order to be more overt about what they were doing and to 'fit things in'. This was most obvious in the case of Ellen throughout, though there was an element of planning and articulation about their plans for all.

Third, by the second stage, all felt the need to exercise greater control over their work and workload. For example, Beth found that it was necessary to 'set personal boundaries' and be much more overt about what the job should entail and what it should not. She felt that it was important to 'clamp down on boundaries and say 'I'm only a lecturer practitioner, I'm not doing such and such', since she saw the overwhelming size of the job as a major reason that people gave when criticizing the role.

Fourth, they assigned priorities to the work. Again, this was especially so for Ellen. She and Felicity (who also talked about assigning priority to different aspects at different times), suggested that when they were very busy 'the ward was the first thing to go'. Conversely, for Ann and Beth, it tended to be the ward work that had to take priority over other activities at times.

Fifth, they had to accept that some aspects of the job would not get done, either at a particular stage or at all, or were in some way controlled. Research was one such activity that was 'temporarily shelved' for all but Ellen. In addition, after the first stage all four used the strategy of 'taking steps to limit their involvement' in certain activities. For example, Ann consciously had to limit the amount of clinical work she did, Beth decided to give up the chairmanship of the Assessment of Practice Group, and Ellen accepted that during this time she was only 'able to do her priority' tasks.

Sixth, during the second stage, a new strategy employed was that of reconceptualizing part of the role. This was especially so for Ellen and to a limited extent for Felicity too. Thus, since Ellen was unable actually to give clinical care she considered her 'clinical practice' responsibility to be 'anything that counts as clinical practice *development*' – in other words, she held a new concept of clinical practice. Similarly, Felicity considered that 'being available to respond to queries or management problems for the ward' was now part of her 'clinical remit'. Thus, she appeared to have broadened her concept of clinical work.

In respect of those aspects where they were dependent (or partially so) on others, for Ann and Beth, much of their work was aimed towards the development of their staff to expand their roles managerially, clinically and as educators and facilitators of others – as Ann said 'to accept some of the ward sister's responsibilities'. Also, by the second stage, all were beginning to develop staff nurses as mentors for the students, not just because they saw it as part of the staff nurses' role to be mentors, but because they recognized that it would be impossible for them to mentor the students themselves to any great extent. This was related to delegation. To some extent they were able to delegate tasks to other people, especially the ward staff, though this was dependent upon the capabilities and availability of staff. Also Beth and Ann were 'greatly helped' by the appointment of a part-time secretary to assist with administrative tasks.

All the lecturer practitioners made efforts to work out the role for themselves and negotiate the role with others (for example, all had meetings with their service and education managers and sometimes with senior colleagues). However, the need to establish professional boundaries was much greater for Ellen, Felicity and David, since all were in a 'collegiate' relationship, rather than having designated managerial responsibilities at the outset.

In relation to the conditions that were deemed necessary for the role, all were concerned with the part they could play in developing a clinical area that would provide good clinical care and at the same time be a suitable learning environment for students. They used such strategies as looking at the staffing structure and skill mix, and devoting time to the development of the staff. There were also important considerations to do with the responsibility attached to the role and the size of the Unit to be managed. In this respect, Beth explicitly linked the issue of viability of the job to responsibility. She had two wards within her remit and considered that in part her job 'worked' because she could concentrate on one ward whilst 'devoting just some time to [the other]'. For her it was an important condition of viability, and she suggested that 'if you have the right size Unit and responsibility, [the job] is not too much'. Conversely, Ellen experienced pressures when her responsibility was extended to a large Unit.

Conclusions from the in-depth study regarding the viability of the job

It appears that Ann recognized the job as being potentially too large, but by the use of various strategies she was able to cope. First, she expanded the amount of time available by consistently working long hours, especially in the first two stages. Second, she redefined the role in such a way as to limit it; for example, she accepted that the amount of clinical work had to diminish, and she found strategies for controlling the students' access when she was working on the ward, such as getting them to book appointments. Third, she managed to 'pass on' some aspects of the job, such as administrative work, to a secretary and facets of the ward management to staff nurses. And fourth, she changed or modified her standards, or compromised. For example, she acknowledged that it was not possible for her to work as a primary nurse very often because of the lack of continuity and the interruptions; she accepted that she could not spend as much time with her ward staff as she wished; she did not attend all the 'Poly' meetings that she might otherwise have felt obliged to (such as Joint Committee); and she did not work clinically with students 'as much as [she] would have liked'.

Whilst Beth also saw the job as potentially too big, she said that, except at times of pressure, she did not experience it as too large. In the main, she viewed this as a concern of others rather than her own. However, she adopted similar strategies to Ann to ensure that the job was manageable. For example, she also worked long hours, especially in the first two stages, and she redefined the role. Thus she set boundaries about what she could and could not do as a lecturer practitioner. Third, just as Ann, she delegated aspects of the job to a secretary and staff nurses. And fourth, she modified her standards by, for example, not working very often as a primary nurse because of the lack of time.

Clearly one of the main reasons that Charlotte did not stay in the job was that she did not find it viable. She considered that the size of the job was a problem, and felt it would have become even more of an issue had she stayed into the second stage. Nevertheless, she did take certain actions in order to try to make the job more possible: for example, she conceded that it was more appropriate to work shifts rather than straight days; she accepted that it was not possible to work as extensively as planned in the role of primary nurse, and she attempted – unsuccessfully – to resolve a difficult relationship with a senior manager. This took place in a context in which Charlotte did not view herself as 'operating as a proper lecturer practitioner' but as someone who was 'mainly preparing the ground for the future'.

David experienced the job as too large. He was expected to take on work that he considered was not part of the role, such as extensive and regular clinical practice 'as a pair of hands', and this was exacerbated by the lack of role clarity both in terms of his own perceptions and the expectations of others. In addition, lack of support from (senior) colleagues was a difficulty and, despite his attempts to tackle the issues, they, along with personal considerations, led to his resignation.

Ellen always considered that the job was too large, and this remained a 'major issue' for her at the end. Another unresolved concern was that of 'balancing the workload' which she spent a great deal of time doing throughout. Her ability to cope and to balance the workload were affected – both positively and negatively – by four types of extraneous factors: the changing personnel occupying the senior nurse post and the nature of her collegiate relationship with that post; the appointment of a ward sister which decreased her original ward responsibilities; undertaking a higher degree with the time pressures this entailed, but also the advantages in terms of the requirement to do clinical research; and the increasing size of the clinical unit within which she had a remit. Nevertheless, the approaches she used to make the job workable included: consistently working long hours; regularly setting priorities, planning and reviewing her time and workload; and not undertaking certain parts of the job at times, but ensuring that 'over a year [she] made a stab at all aspects of the job'. She also reconceptualized aspects of the job so that they were more possible, for example, by viewing her clinical responsibilities as less to do with working clinically and more to do with working intermittently with nurses and providing clinical support and advice. Linked with this, she modified her aspirations about what was possible to achieve, especially in relation to the clinical component.

It appears that Felicity, in common with Ann and Beth, saw the job as being potentially too large, and during the fieldwork she experienced it as such. Nevertheless, she took similar steps to her colleagues to ameliorate this. For example, she, too, consistently worked long hours, and redefined the role; for example, she accepted that the amount of clinical work and activities had to be limited to an average of one or two days a week and that she could not be responsible for the day-to-day clinical work of the ward. Also, she found strategies for tackling her difficulties in turning down those wishing her to do more things. Third, she persuaded other nurses to undertake aspects of the job, such as facets of the ward work (e.g. preparation of dependency figures and collection of SDU information). And fourth, she gave up some aspects of the job altogether, such as attendance at certain of the committee meetings.

In addition, the viability of the job for Felicity was not only to do with the size of the job and the amount of time available. There were also issues to do with the nature of her role *vis-à-vis* the ward sister role and another senior sister role, which at the outset and to a certain extent later affected her ability to exercise the kind of authority that she considered was necessary for the job. However, by the final stage she suggested that this had largely been clarified and resolved, in part by her working through them and in part by organizational changes and the introduction of new systems for resource management.

In conclusion, the job of lecturer practitioner was clearly experienced as too large, or seen as potentially too great. The ability to cope with the varying pressures over time, and the issues of the need to balance workload and to set and review priorities were common. However, the need to clarify the authority of the role, to work out and negotiate relationships with senior colleagues, and to decide on what was appropriate and possible in terms of the clinical component of the role were more relevant to individuals rather than to all. A number of common strategies were employed to develop the role and ensure that it was feasible. Nevertheless, although clarification, reconceptualization and delegation had long-term advantages for the viability of the job, setting priorities, forward planning and compromising on the activities of the role were all aspects that needed frequent review, and working long hours was considered by the lecturer practitioners to be undesirable over a long period of time.

The unified nature of the role

The research focused on whether or not the LP was perceived and experienced as a unified role in their terms. If not, was this seen as problematic and in need of resolution? In the beginning, the pattern for at least four out of five (less so for Charlotte) was that of a large number of separate activities. Indeed, Ann and Beth in particular distinguished clinical work from 'Poly' work or talked about 'clinical and education activities'. Ellen, too, made a large number of distinctions between different aspects of her role – more than any of the others, and David referred quite specifically to the tutoring work as being separate from clinical and other aspects.

None the less, Ellen talked about the activities 'overlapping in reality'. In addition she saw it as part of her job 'to help others understand the concept of the unified whole'. Also, Ann and Beth had a notion of a 'central core' to the job. Beth described the 'great strength of the role as . . . pivotal on the nature of the nursing care' and she saw the clinical work as central to the job in order to improve care *and* prepare the ward for the students coming. Similarly, Ann talked about 'working on the ward' and 'caring for patients' as the 'keystone' or 'crux' of everything she was trying to do as a lecturer practitioner, with 'staff development being integral to [her] ward work', and with all of this paving the way for and contributing towards the development of a good clinical environment in which students could learn. She reinforced the role as one job by saying: 'I think you need a holistic approach [to the job] and every facet . . . is important; one bit without another bit just doesn't work.'

Conversely, Felicity described most of her job as 'being on the ward or to do with the ward', but other activities, such as attending student presentations and module development, were 'bits of the role that [she] could not actually unify with the ward', thus 'making [her] unsure about the idea of a unified role'.

In the next two stages, though the pattern of quite distinct and separate activities was still apparent, all four were talking about 'the integrated nature of the job'. For Ellen, this appeared to be about the many functions that any one activity could have – for example, a conversation with a staff nurse could be for the personal benefit of that nurse, part of mentor preparation, and indirectly be contributing to student learning. Similarly, Beth talked about the different parts as being 'closely intertwined' – and the distinction between practice, education and other aspects *per se* as being very unclear.

Likewise, Ann argued that her job was 'unified' in three inter-related ways – through the possession of authority, a common aim and a single location. She suggested that as a lecturer practitioner who was also the senior nurse, she had the authority for clinical practice, staff development, management *and* student education, and she referred to everything she did as being aimed towards a common end, and within one location saying:

I think it's a new job – the whole idea of lecturer practitioner is facilitating learning by focusing on the ward – you don't leave the ward for teaching. And everything you do is for Poly *and* service; it shouldn't be divided.

For Felicity, the notion of integration was in part to do with location ('the job started to become more integrated . . . when the students hit the ward and I was on the ward nearly all the time') and in part, her perception of the relationship of different aspects – 'I began to see how the bits fitted together . . . and the whole role made more sense to me'.

Conclusions regarding the unified nature of the role

In conclusion, no understanding was generated about the perception of Charlotte and David in relation to unification. However, it appears that all the other four did perceive their roles as unified despite the pattern being one of many separate activities. Unification seemed to have two main meanings for them. First, and most pervasively, it meant that whilst their jobs comprised a number of facets – notably clinical, managerial, educational and staff development – when they were undertaking any one activity it was often conceived as comprising a combination of two or more of the facets, and was multi-purpose. For example, the activity was aimed at providing care for patients, facilitating staff development *and* paving the way for students. The term 'integrated' was often used in this respect.

The second way in which three out of the four seemed to conceive the role as unified was through the notion of the role having a clinical core, with all the other activities related to, or emanating from, this core. In part, there was a geographical element to this; they were 'firmly based in clinical settings' and saw the other activities (for example, the educational aspects) as primarily taking place in that clinical setting.

The different LP models

Ann and Beth both referred to being in the 'pure model' whereby they were senior sisters for a unit, ward sister for one of the wards and lecturer practitioner. Beth felt that this model was being promoted by the Polytechnic rather than the others, and Ann stated that in her mind it was 'the only *true* lecturer practitioner model'. Ellen quite specifically saw herself in a different model, and one where she was 'in a collegiate relationship' with her Senior Nurse.

On the other hand, David did not liken his role to any particular model, though he did compare his role with that of 'a clinical practice development nurse' in that he 'kept an eye on what the staff were doing and gave them ideas' for developing their practice. He felt this could be rationalized in terms of 'developing the learning environment so that it would be suitable for Poly students'. Similarly, Charlotte saw herself not adhering to a model, but operating much more as a clinically-based Senior Nurse. She played down her role as lecturer practitioner – which she seemed to view as someone with a tutor's qualification.

Felicity considered her 'model' of lecturer practitioner to be different from all of the four stated in the plans, though it appears that she wished to align it to the fourth model, the collegiate role. This was in part to do with the particular circumstances of the post (i.e. having an established ward sister in post in the ward where she was based, and another senior sister), and in part because of the initial confusion and lack of clarity over the nature of her role and relationship with these other roles. Since initially she was 'not able to operate the model in the way [she] would like' this gave rise to 'challenges'.

During the second stage, Ann – for practical reasons and through her knowledge and observation of other lecturer practitioners – conceded that other models might be both necessary and workable. She suggested that whilst 'her model' was the best, there were not likely to be enough 'suitable' people to fill the roles. But from her own experience, the one principle she felt should not be compromised was that of power and authority, because she did not want 'to lose the notion that the LP is accountable for the areas that she places students in'. However, in expanding this view later, she considered it was important to balance principles with pragmatics, saying:

> Whilst I still believe you need power and authority in your own area, ... when you're placing students on wards that aren't your own, I don't think you can be responsible for them. Yet there aren't enough places to always put them where the LP can guarantee the standards of practice.

At the final stage, neither Ann nor Beth seemed to see their particular model of lecturer practitioner as an issue meriting much attention. It did not seem to be problematic and was not mentioned. When questioned, Ellen did not see her role as fitting the original models. In fact, she considered that it was unhelpful to think of the role in terms of a model at all. As she argued:

> I don't think about it like that [as to whether it fits a model]. I think of the principles. I didn't even look at the original models.

As far as I am concerned I think that the role I am in achieves the principles that were originally put out as the lecturer practitioner role, and I stand by those. There are definitely different ways of doing it, but the focus should be on the principles not the models. [In this respect] having core sections in a job description is good.

However, she did distinguish between her role – which she described as 'combined' – and the 'all-in-one role', that is, the pure model, and suggested that workload was a particular issue in the latter. She further identified the problem of other people's perceptions of the role, 'since all the LP posts [in the health authority] are different', yet share the same principle, notably authority at a senior level. She compared this particular health authority's lecturer practitioners with those elsewhere 'where the principles are very different'.

Felicity, too, still did not see her role as fitting into one of the four models – even though 'senior managers were trying to slot [her] in' – yet she did not reject the notion of different models. As she said: 'I'm told it's model 4, but it's a "cuckoo-in-the-nest" model, plonked on top of what's there'. In responding to the researcher's account, she explained this further, saying: 'I don't think there is anybody else who has been put in on top of the establishment and then taken on the resource issues, though I may be wrong.' Additionally, she considered that her managerial authority did not become absolutely clear to others until she took on the role of SDU manager for the ward. At this point, she felt that she was able to operate the role in the way she saw it should be, and that it was not really a problem any longer. However, there was a residual issue to do with the extent to which she should, and would, intervene with staff on the ward who were in potentially stressful situations, given the existence of a ward sister with responsibilities in relation to ward staff.

Conclusions regarding role differentiation

Ann described her role as the pure model from the outset and, whilst she believed it to be the most appropriate, she conceded that for pragmatic reasons it may be necessary to have other approaches to the role also. She always felt clear about the differentiation between lecturer practitioner jobs, clinical teachers and joint appointments, distinguishing them in terms of the authority accruing to lecturer practitioners, and the integrated nature of the lecturer practitioner role, and considered that this should be conveyed to others. Essentially, neither the model she occupied, nor its comparison with other roles, was problematic to her. Similarly, Beth promoted her role as preferential, but this was never a major consideration for her, and neither was its comparison with other roles.

By contrast, Charlotte did not consider herself as a 'standard' lecturer practitioner, but more of a Senior Nurse with 'some responsibilities to pave the way for the students'. She had an initial conception that all lecturer practitioners would be the same, that is, clinically based practitioners and teachers. However, her experience suggested that there were many different versions, including, by her implication, some who were much less clinically oriented.

David drew a comparison between his role and that of a clinical practice development nurse, both perceiving the job to be described as such in the job specification, and to be like it in practice. However, he appeared to be ambivalent about this, and somewhat unclear about what his role should actually be. It remained an issue and was one of the factors leading to his resignation.

Ellen found the concept of different models unhelpful and preferred to base the development of her role on the idea of a set of principles. She did, however, contrast her role with others described as 'all-in-one' roles. She suggested that because of the breadth of workload her role was preferable, and the other was 'difficult to sustain' and likely to lead to burnout. An outstanding concern for her was the understanding of others about the particular lecturer practitioner concept in the health authority where, she argued, there were many versions but a common issue – that of a certain level of authority held by all senior nurses.

The nature of Felicity's role, and the fact that it did not adhere to a particular model, was problematic to her in that she had to cope with a situation that was sensitive, and one where her role was overlaid on others. She had to do a great deal of clarification, but it seems that eventually the main issues were resolved to her satisfaction. She accepted that her model was necessarily a hybrid, but a largely workable one.

In conclusion, it appears that three out of the six lecturer practitioners – occupying two types of role – promoted their 'model' or approach as either preferable to or more viable than the alternative. Two either did not see themselves as lecturer practitioners in the same way as others, or likened their role to another role. The sixth, whilst accepting that she was in a different role, worked at overcoming some of the problems inherent in the job. All four in the final stage were convinced that being a lecturer practitioner was different from alternative roles, such as clinical teachers and joint appointments. They said it was different, felt it to be different, and identified the distinctions as being the authority in the role and 'the generation of the role' from a particular practice setting. However, it remained unclear whether there were further distinguishing factors beyond these.

The viability as seen by the survey LPs

The survey LPs were asked about the viability of their role with the following results (percentages indicate those ticking this category):

The LP role is:
- a workable role all of the time (7%)
- a workable role most of the time (27%)
- workable, but only under certain conditions or by using particular strategies (60%)
- not workable at all (2%)

The strategies used to make the job possible were:
- working to priorities (95%)
- regularly working longer hours than they were contracted for (91%)
- not doing parts of the role (55%)
- delegating parts of the role to others (51%)
- having colleagues who voluntarily shared the work (47%).

In addition, the survey LPs mentioned as important factors: the need to manage time well; learning to say 'no'; having supportive colleagues and managers; and having secretarial help. It was evident therefore that there was considerable similarity between the six LPs and the survey LPs in terms of working long hours and working to priorities, but a more variable pattern in relation to other strategies. Some lecturer practitioners added here that there was no one to delegate aspects of their role to, or that they had 'no suitable colleagues to share the work with'. The point was also made that this was not a static situation and that 'sometimes [they] decided that they could not do parts of the role temporarily when other things had to take priority'.

Survey LPs' views of the model

Survey LPs were asked about the appropriateness of their particular model. Responses indicated that 40% felt that their model of lecturer practitioner had more advantages than disadvantages; 31% considered that their model had some advantages and some disadvantages; 11% suggested their model to be ideal or very appropriate; 4% thought that it had more disadvantages than advantages, and 7% that it was flawed or unworkable. (Four people gave other answers.)

A number of advantages for the different models were outlined and the following percentages of survey LPs indicated these to be the case for their model:

- having authority for clinical practice (73%)
- being able to share the managerial responsibility in a collegiate relationship (42%)
- not having the burden of being a senior nurse/ward sister as well as being an LP (40%).
- being the manager of a clinical area (38%)
- having clarity between this and other roles (38%).

A number of disadvantages – actual or potential – of the models occupied were also evident, as follows:

- having too many responsibilities in one role (58%)
- having a lack of clarity between their role and other people's in the clinical area (33%)
- having another manager in the clinical area, confusing the role (25%)
- not having sufficient authority for clinical practice (25%)
- not being able to share the managerial authority (15%)
- not being the manager of the clinical area (13%)
- having the burden of being senior nurse/ward sister as well as LP (11%).

In summary, the LPs in the in-depth study and nearly three-quarters of all survey lecturer practitioners suggested that 'having authority for clinical practice' was an advantage, and in line with this, a quarter found insufficient authority for clinical practice to be a problem. Thus, authority for clinical practice is clearly an important issue for many lecturer practitioners. Furthermore, having role clarity was seen as positive by a significant proportion, and this was matched by a similar percentage who found lack of role clarity a disadvantage. However, just as in the in-depth study, there was a division of opinion over the aspect of being manager as well as an LP. Whilst 40% of lecturer practitioners felt that being a manager of a clinical area was an advantage and 13% identified lack of managerial authority as being a disadvantage, a similar proportion of lecturer practitioners (38%) welcomed 'not having the burden of being a senior nurse/ward sister as well as being an LP', with 11% feeling that 'having the burden of being senior nurse/ward sister as well as LP' was a concern. This latter finding is supported by the fairly high proportion of lecturer practitioners (42%) who felt it to be an advantage that they could share the managerial responsibility in a collegiate relationship, as well as the 11% who wished that they could be in a collegiate relationship.

Problems identified by survey LPs

The viability of the role is clearly related to the problems and challenges found within the role. Survey LPs were asked to identify what these were. They appeared to be related to a number of different aspects of the job such as: the size, breadth and demands of the job (e.g. time and workload); the role relationships (e.g. expectations of others, working with students, mentors, staff, other managers and other professionals); the nature of the role (e.g. clinical practice, education, authority, responsibilities, management, the balance of all these and conflicting demands); the effects of the job on the person (e.g. effect on personal life and stress); and contextual factors (such as the Polytechnic/University department and resources).

Size, breadth and demands of job

By far the most frequent type of response concerned the problem of 'time in general'. Over a quarter of lecturer practitioners (17 or 31%) mentioned this as a major concern. Six used the term 'time management', and others talked about 'time constraints', 'working long hours', 'fitting everything in' and 'containing projects within the time available'. However, these comments appeared to be couched in terms of a challenge rather than a problem, and there was not the negative feel to them as conveyed by other responses such as: 'too much to do in too little time', 'never enough time to do all', 'not enough time to do the job properly', 'trying not to survive merely by working overtime' and 'coping with long hours'.

In addition, 13 (24%) respondents specified what they wanted more time for, or the implications for them of this lack of time. They required 'time for . . .' 'keeping students well supported', 'focusing in-depth on several projects and not just one', 'reading', 'preparation for teaching', 'curriculum development', 'evaluation of clinical work', 'meetings', 'completion of all the education aspects', 'nursing patients', 'being effective in the clinical area managerially and clinically', and 'to write about my work and share with others'. Others focused specifically on the lack of 'time for research or for personal development' or for themselves.

Six lecturer practitioners (11%) referred to the related problem of 'workload' in the sense of 'having too many demands', and needing to 'cope with the volume of work'. In addition, workload was also linked with two other types of responses, the concern of one lecturer practitioner about the 'size of the job' ('being a senior nurse and an LP – the role is too large. I haven't been able to do either role as I would like'), and the 'ability to say no', which two lecturer practitioners mentioned ('saying "no", especially when projects are interesting' and 'learning to say no without feeling guilty'). Further, two were worried about 'standards' because of their workload and the size of the role, expressing their concerns as: 'achieving my workload to a consistently high standard in all spheres' and more generally 'maintaining standards'. And in a related point, another lecturer practitioner found 'having to compromise to achieve [her] aims' to be a problem.

Role relationships

Over a quarter of all respondents were concerned about 'expectations and role relationships'. Sixteen lecturer practitioners (29%) talked about the expectations of other people, and the problem of 'meeting expectations', 'pleasing all people all or even some of the time', 'being able to fulfil customers and students at all times', 'satisfying demands of ward staff who want you 100% ward based', 'clinical colleagues who see me as manager; they forget the other bits' and the 'need to constantly reinforce the importance of clinical obligations to education colleagues'. Role relationships was another issue: for example, 'the difficulty of being accepted by a resistant team of sisters, and the undermining of my credibility by devious means', 'hostility from senior nursing staff in this Centre', 'feeling of resentment and desertion on part of some colleagues now I'm not so much in the clinical area' and 'integrating my role with other existing senior roles'.

Whereas a very high proportion of the lecturer practitioners had found 'students' to be a positive aspect of the role, three identified difficulties in this respect, citing as concerns 'ensuring students receive the best possible clinical experience in the practice area', 'being able to give students the level of support I would like' and 'coping with students' lack of enthusiasm and insight'. Likewise, although 'working with mentors and staff nurses' was a satisfaction for many, a small minority (three) raised issues such as 'supporting and developing mentors', and 'the stress of asking for mentors' as well as 'maintaining the emotional energy to support staff nurses'.

There was also a related physical concern, that of 'geographical isolation' from colleagues. Three lecturer practitioners talked about 'loss of geographically close peers', 'the difficulty of looking after personal tutees 25 miles away' and 'the lack of communication with peers who are physically distanced'. A further individual referred to the general problem of 'communication': 'difficulties of negotiation, liaison and communication with all'.

The intrinsic nature of the role

There were problems to do with the overall nature of the role, such as the extent of its clarity, and how the different aspects did or did not fit together. Thus, ten lecturer practitioners (18%) were concerned about the lack of 'role clarity' or ambiguity about their roles. An equal number of responses (10 or 18%) referred to the problem of 'balance' within the job. Eight actually used this term: for example, 'balancing everything' and 'balancing priorities', as well as 'juggling time, getting the service/education balance right'. Others described it as 'dividing myself and time fairly and equally between two jobs', and 'managing the needs of two large institutions'.

Another very similar category to balance was the problem of 'conflicting demands', which received eight mentions (15%). This was variously described as: 'being pulled in different directions – staff nurses, students, surgeons, patients all need you', 'conflicting demands of service and education; you are needed on the ward to cover sickness, but also have 12 essays to mark by a deadline', and 'being torn between education and practice (clinical usually loses)'. Others referred to 'having a primary role with caseload and trying to develop and extend practice', 'staying in contact with reality (nursing practice) and not becoming too academic', 'the difficulty of maintaining the whole role with clinical pressures', and 'the split [between education and service] is difficult to manage, giving conflict and overload'.

Three further categories were linked with this – the fragmentation of the role, integrating parts of the role and having two bosses. Respondents talked about the problem of 'spreading [themselves] too thin, not doing anything well, being neither expert in education nor practice' and 'feeling fragmented, jack of all trades, master of none'. Some were concerned about 'integration', 'trying to marry both halves of the job' and 'helping others see it's an integrated role with practice as the focus'. (Conversely, a very much higher proportion of lecturer practitioners – over a quarter – had viewed the ability to integrate or combine education and practice as a positive feature of the job.) In addition, two were concerned about 'having two bosses with different aims' and 'the frustration of accountability to two managers (education and service) with different priorities'.

In addition, individual parts of the job, such as clinical practice, were an issue. In terms of this, six lecturer practitioners raised various points. For example, one talked about 'the lack of clinical practice [in her job], resulting in reduced competence and credibility' and similarly, one mentioned that her clinical role had changed from when she was a sister: as she said 'I am not able to be primary nurse as I was when a sister'. Another 'felt guilty that her clinical area was not perfect', and one that she had difficulty in 'developing a theoretical basis for nursing in her area'. One respondent considered that 'one clinical area only is sufficient for the role', the implication being that her role was overloaded with responsibility for more than one clinical area. Finally, one suggested that 'practice [in her area] was not valued as it should be within the curriculum'. (In addition, another lecturer practitioner suggested that 'lack of continuity of the clinical work' was a frustration.)

Another aspect of the role that was deemed problematic by six lecturer practitioners (11%) was that of 'authority'. Two mentioned that they had 'no authority in reality', the implication being that although there was authority in theory, this was not actually the case. The other four talked more specifically about the problem of authority in respect of particular parts of their roles; for example, they saw as a difficulty 'authority in the clinical area, and not being allowed in', 'undermining of authority on educational issues' and 'having little managerial authority for clinical practice and learning environment means I carry very little clout'. (In another category, where authority was not specifically mentioned, but the principle was clearly there, 'responsibility for the learning environment' was clearly an issue. Thus, two lecturer practitioners identified as problematic 'having education responsibility for another clinical area for which I have no other links or responsibilities', and 'lack of control over the learning environment'.)

Linked with this was the issue of credibility. Whereas two lecturer practitioners had found enhanced clinical credibility to be a positive feature of their roles, three others found 'gaining credibility' a difficulty. This was evidenced by their comments: 'updating, being there, thus gaining credibility with both organizations', 'trying to get the "street cred" right in the clinical areas' and 'lack of clinical practice, resulting in reduced competence and credibility'.

Finally, the ability of the lecturer practitioners to achieve development was also a concern. Although 'development' was cited as a positive feature of the role for a number of the lecturer practitioners, conversely it was also seen as a problem, albeit by relatively few people. Thus four mentioned as a concern 'developing practice', as evidenced by the following comments: 'maintaining enthusiasm and motivation for a sustained period of time for developing the ward and staff' and 'trying to develop a new service whilst myself needing induction'. Three found the 'development of the role' problematic, with one using this term, another talking about 'developing the role and being organized', and a third, 'developing a workable role by developing another colleague as LP and changing the concept of practice to research practice'. A third notion of development was that of 'self-development', whereby three respondents outlined concerns of 'building up confidence as manager and educator', 'developing a new service whilst [at the same time] myself needing induction', and 'helping peers to develop and finding someone to develop me'.

Effects of the job on the person

There were two concerns that appeared to be related, the first about the 'effects of work on personal life', and the second on 'stress'. Five lecturer practitioners referred to the problem of 'the job affecting life outside work', 'the long hours [needed] both at work and home trying to get work done' and 'working long hours, with little time for anything else'. One talked about having difficulty 'relaxing when off duty' and another, 'maintaining life outside work and sanity'. The implications of these comments is that of personal pressure, and four respondents specifically referred to this by mentioning 'the burn-out factor', 'keeping up the pace – you can't go on for ever', 'the difficulty of controlling the stress levels of the job' and 'looking after myself – the job is stressful'.

In a linked theme, three respondents mentioned the 'loneliness' of the job, and the lack of guidelines – 'there are few guidelines or support, it's lonely', 'the loneliness [is a problem], we no longer have a paediatric team', and 'it is a lonely job, and there is need for peer support'. This appeared to be an emotional concern.

Context

Six lecturer practitioners found a factor outside of the role itself as problematic – the 'Polytechnic (University) department'. Two had difficulty in understanding the system ('trying to explain the Poly system to clinical staff when I don't understand it myself' and 'the gobbledygook of the Poly system'), and in a similar point, one had problems 'seeing the nursing degree holistically'. For another, the concern was to do with 'keeping up-to-date with the running of [the department], both undergraduate and post graduate courses', and one did not 'feel part of the department'. Finally, one lecturer practitioner cited two problems in relation to the department – a 'disproportionate sharing of the work in the department' alongside 'unresolved organizational and political problems', though the nature of these problems was not specified.

Interestingly, resources were little mentioned specifically as an issue, except for the 'lack of clerical or secretarial support' by four lecturer practitioners. Two stated the problem in this way, one specifically referring to the 'lack of clerical support in the clinical area' and another, 'the lack of adequate resources, but especially secretarial support'.

Viability of the job from the perspectives of mentors and team leaders, students, educators and managers

Finally the perspectives of others were interesting as far as the viability of the LP role was concerned. All the mentors and team leaders in the interview study agreed that it was a very large role, a 'huge job', and that their lecturer practitioner always 'seemed to be very busy'. However, the extent to which this was seen as problematic varied across the group. Again, this appeared to be related primarily though not entirely to the particular lecturer practitioner, and certainly to the kind of responsibility they held. Thus, with Ann, whilst she was described as 'putting in a lot of hours', this was not talked about as a problem for her as such. Rather, the job itself was considered to be 'in theory unmanageable', or a role which had 'become too big with too many expectations'. Nevertheless, respondents articulated the way in which Ann had managed the job to make it work.

> The answer to having too much clinical responsibility is to do what Ann did which was to hand a lot of responsibilities to the ward team e.g. the day-to-day management of the ward, off duty, annual leave. This relieved her of the responsibilities and encouraged the ward team to take them on, whilst recognizing the limitations that they have to work within.

> Ann showed ways in which you can develop people to help in the role, and imbued them with a sense of ownership and self-confidence, so they can start taking some of the load.

For Ellen, there was a difference of opinion. Whilst acknowledging that she was busy, one considered that her job was manageable, but another said:

> She's got the students and she's doing us as well. She spends a lot of time here [on the ward]. Sometimes I get the feeling that she could do with just being LP for students only or LP for the ward.

Similarly, the views about Beth were varied. Whereas one felt her role worked 'as long as people she is working with respect the fact that she has got other things to do', two considered that the role of sister and LP should be separated. As one of these said:

To me an LP should just be LP and not a sister. From their part, I find it hard to believe that they can cope with being sister and an LP. To me they are quite separate roles/jobs. Also, though she's very conscientious, I don't think she gives enough time to the students.

And another:

I think there should be someone more senior to take over on the ward to manage that side of things. Seeing Beth pulled so many ways, I think she could do with some of those responsibilities taken off her shoulders to concentrate on the students. Maybe she could come back to work on the ward two days a week or whatever she wants to do.

In respect of Felicity, there were three different responses. One considered that the 'job was getting bigger all the time', that it was 'a lot of work for one person to do', yet conceded that since all the aspects interlinked it would be difficult to see what Felicity could 'drop realistically and fulfil what was set down on paper'. A second said:

The job in theory is viable and the ideas behind it are brilliant. [Nevertheless], it's trying to get the balance right. She's around for people to know who she is. She's there if I need her, but sometimes I feel she's not here *enough*, her responsibility to the Poly outweighs her responsibility to the ward, and sometimes you don't see her for a week or two. Her Poly commitments are very big. I think the element of practice is too hard for her to do.

And a third suggested that the job should change. As she put it:

Some of the things she does on the ward could be taken over by a nurse manager. Felicity is involved in education but the sort of stuff she is doing on the managerial side, it doesn't necessarily have to be an educator doing that. It could be a senior nurse.

All of the students considered that the job was big, and all but two (one in respect of Ellen and the other, Beth) saw this as a problem or potential problem. In terms of the viability of the job, interestingly four (just over half the group) talked about their awareness of the need 'to get the balance between the parts right', and the possible tensions between the two aspects. Thus as one said: 'I think that maybe a part of their job could suffer because they are trying to do so much.' Another suggested that 'there might be the temptation to spend more than half of one's time on each role, and the workload would become very heavy'. And a third concluded that:

> LPs experience a lot of friction between practising and education in the sense of loyalties to practice placements and loyalties as lecturers. I think they feel they're struggling in two different worlds.

Several argued that the ability to manage the job varied between lecturer practitioners, and cited examples of other lecturer practitioners that they felt had not coped with the workload as well as the four under study.

The educators agreed that the LP role was 'a very big job', but that there were strategies and conditions that could make it viable. For example, two suggested that 'it's a very skilled job that requires critical analysis and goal setting about what you want to achieve', but by doing this it was possible. In addition, one considered that administrative support was important 'to make it an achievable job'. Two pointed out that if the job was thought of as half a sister's role and half a lecturer, then it was not going to work. As one said:

> It has to be more flexible than that. I do think it's possible if team leaders accept that they are the accountable ones for managing their teams and co-operating in managing the ward on a day-to-day basis.

All three talked about the important issue of the different models of lecturer practitioner. Two concurred that the combined senior nurse and LP role was preferable because: 'it gives the accountability and credibility within the clinical area'; 'an LP in this role does not have to work out their authority, they have it by nature of their role', and 'the senior sister can influence direct management policy'. However, both placed riders on this in that one considered that such a role was 'unreasonable to sustain for individuals', and the other, 'that not everyone would want this mega-load'. The third member of the group took the stance that whilst her lecturer practitioner colleague 'had no choice in the model' since there was an existing ward sister in post, this 'threw up major dichotomies', yet the role was made workable by careful, and time-consuming, negotiation and development on the lecturer practitioner's part. All agreed that in practice a range of models would be both necessary and appropriate.

In common with the educators, two of the service managers commented upon the most appropriate model for the lecturer practitioner role, but they were diametrically opposed in their views.

One said that whilst she felt the idea of the lecturer practitioner also being a senior sister was quite good in principle, she did not agree with the combining of the LP and senior nurse role in practice because 'you need extremely different skills to educate and to manage, and it's very difficult to combine those two things in one role'. On the other hand, the other was predisposed to the joint senior nurse and LP role because 'it is the senior sister who sets policy, and this is important', although this respondent did 'admit to being biased by the success of Ann and Beth's roles'.

Conclusion

When comparing the different parts of the research, it is interesting to note the common themes. First, whilst the job of lecturer practitioner was seen by the LPs themselves and others as very large, this was not necessarily conceived of as a problem. Second, it was generally recognized that in order to achieve the principles of the role, various methods had to be used to make the job workable. Finally, and linking the first two points, the role of lecturer practitioner was not deemed as inherently unviable. Rather, it was up to individuals within their different setting, and with the support of others, to negotiate and work out what was necessary, effective and possible. Importantly, this varied between contexts.

Chapter 8

Conclusions and beyond

This final chapter brings together some of the insights gained from the research – the rich, in-depth accounts of the lives of the six LPs, the views of those working closely with them and the responses from the survey of all the LPs, some 55 individuals. In addition, it brings this research up-to-date by reference to a subsequent review of the LP role, as well as considering how these lecturer practitioners fit into the wider context.

First, a number of conclusions can be drawn from the research – five being of particular interest and of relevance to professional education, not just within nursing and midwifery, but also more broadly.

The LP and the politics of professional education

The programme and the plans for lecturer practitioners can be seen to stem from the kind of thinking underpinning that of Judge (1980). In discussing the politics of teacher education, Judge suggested that the teaching profession needed the status of university preparation, but that this training should take place in schools – thus combining the university (academic) status with the practical value of being in schools.

Traditionally, teacher education has tended to have as the focus the college or other higher education institution, with student teachers only going into schools for periods of teaching practice. The same has been true for the training of nurse tutors, but not for the pre-registration education of nurses. Here the emphasis has been on the 'learner' nurse and the apprenticeship model combined with theoretical input within relatively low status schools of nursing. Nevertheless, changes in the organization of nurse education have been aimed at establishing a model which is much more akin to traditional teacher education – with 'student' nurses who are primarily supernumerary and Colleges of Nursing and Midwifery which are now largely part of higher education.

Alongside the increasing academic recognition of nursing as a whole has been an increasing acceptance of the importance of nursing experience and 'practice-centred' nurse education (UKCC, 1986). However, it seems that in Project 2000 these two strands could easily be in tension, with the 'academic' study of nursing taking place in the College or academic department under the tutelage of the 'tutors' (or more likely 'lecturers') and the practice of nursing being within wards and clinical areas under the guidance of ward sisters and staff nurses, with no organizational link between the two. Similarly, in this study the degree course comprised theoretical modules based in the academic institution and practice modules, entirely led and run by lecturer practitioners, in clinical settings. But, it was argued in the plans that practice had been hitherto down-valued, and that it should be central to the programme. Thus the lecturer practitioners – with their practice and education remit, and their high status in both the education and practice realms – were deemed to be critical in the move towards academic recognition of nursing and a greater valuing of practice in the education of the student nurses. In effect, they provided this necessary organizational link.

Therefore, it is suggested that, viewed in political and organizational terms, the lecturer practitioner role can be seen as an appropriate way of resolving the tension inherent in the desire to combine the academic status with a clinical base. Lecturer practitioners can be perceived as credible lecturers and practitioners with authority in both arenas. This in turn is related to the role of the lecturer practitioner in respect of theory and practice.

Combining practice and education: theory–practice tensions

The rationales for a new role which combined responsibilities for practice and education were various and mostly to do with improving nurse education. Thus, this combination was considered beneficial in a number of ways. For example, it was deemed to enhance the integration of theory and practice, to rectify the situation whereby practice has been consistently undervalued in nurse education and to raise the status of clinical practice to equivalence with (or even superiority over) the theoretical contribution, given the growing recognition of the complexities of practice. Furthermore, it was hoped that it would attract people who, as experienced educators and practitioners, had the ability to theorize about and analyse nursing practice, and who would necessarily enhance standards of practice and provide a better educational environment.

Closely linked with this was the view that the lecturer practitioner role was there specifically to solve a problem of theory and practice. This was the conventional one – experienced in educational programmes for most professions – of a lack of easy consistency or connectedness between the ideas taught in the classroom (theory) and the things done or observed in the wards (practice). Traditionally, solving this problem presumes not only the (above mentioned) better integration of the two, or the 'bridging of the gap', but also the putting of theory into practice, with the lecturer practitioner as a key facilitator of the process.

Cutting across these sentiments the plans demonstrated there to be other ambitious ideas – about the nature of good nursing, and the need to move from task-centred to patient-centred nursing, with the rejection of a 'medical model' of nursing for a concept of nursing with its own discipline. In addition, there were views on the nature of professional knowledge, with questions being raised in the name of Schön (1983) and Benner (1984) in respect of the value of the theory-into-practice technicist view of nursing knowledge, and an espousal of reflective practitioner ideals and associated notions of theory being derived from practice. Nevertheless, whilst the ideals of reflection were embodied in the concept of lecturer practitioner, they appear to have been construed as meaning encountering in the course of practice phenomena that could be understood in terms of the theoretical ideas which had previously been taught.

The findings of the research clearly showed there to be an unresolved theory–practice problem. First, there was the vagueness on the part of the lecturer practitioners themselves, and the lack of shared understandings on the part of others relating to them, about the issues. Second, it seemed that the criteria of lecturers, mentors and lecturer practitioners, where they were evident, were not always aligned, and groups such as students did not always see the point of certain aspects, for example, reflection on practice in terms of theory. Further, there were still tensions between what 'should be happening' and what was actually happening; for a variety of reasons what was being taught in the course did not necessarily match with the reality of practice. Finally, there was the tension between assessment of good practice and talk of good practice; the learning contracts focused on reflection on practice, leaving the question as to whether this truly indicated the quality of students' practice.

There were instances where lecturer practitioners were addressing these issues; for example: by trying to develop practice so that it more nearly matched their notions of what it should be about;

by themselves acting as exemplars or role models for mentors; or by 'theorizing' about practice when in an assessment situation. However, it can be argued that even if there had been more emphasis in the actions of the lecturer practitioners themselves on the derivation of theory from practice, as espoused in the more recent literature, to some extent in the plans and in the rhetoric of the lecturer practitioners, this is likely to have been equally inadequate.

It would appear that the traditional theory-into-practice notion as a basis for the concept of lecturer practitioner as well as the contemporary ideas of developing theory from practice are both problematic. Rafferty *et al.* (1996) made a persuasive case that 'a gap between theory and practice is not only inevitable but necessary for change to occur in nursing education', that theory and practice should 'be held in dynamic tension for clinical creativity to develop', and that this tension can be usefully exploited in teaching and research. They argued that

> as Kuhn (1962) suggests that scientific revolutions occur by the generation of anomalies which cannot be accommodated within the existing research paradigm, so might it be with the theory/practice gap. Rather than eliminating it, we need to encourage a contradictory dialectic between theory and practice. (Rafferty et al., 1996, p. 689)

It seems both inevitable and appropriate that theory and practice should be thought of as different parts of the whole which is nursing – each important in its own right – and without the necessity for theory to be imposed on practice or alternatively practice to dictate theory. Evidence, especially from the in-depth study, suggests that lecturer practitioners were in some measure getting to grips with such issues, were challenging the assumption that their task was a simple one of transmitting a known body of 'proven' knowledge into the practice of nursing, and were recognizing the complexity of the theory–practice interface. None the less, a problem remained, seemingly because neither the lecturer practitioners nor the scheme as a whole had coherent ideas of theory practice relationships, and therefore lecturer practitioners had no clear way of defining their role in this respect.

In conclusion, it can be argued that the lecturer practitioner role is actually and potentially powerful in promoting the dialectic between the theory and practice. In turn, this might be seen as a major part of, or extrapolation from, the 'management of learning' role which can be viewed as a major step forward offered by the lecturer practitioner scheme.

Being an educational manager of practice

Explicit also in this scheme is that of the lecturer practitioner as a educational manager of practice. Although in looking at the plans for lecturer practitioners there was no clear articulation of their role as educational managers of practice, it was strikingly evident from the observation of their practice that they were acting as managers of educational environments and student learning rather than as 'hands-on' teachers. It seems that the reason for this was that it presented a solution to a number of the problems and challenges that the lecturer practitioners were confronted with. For example, it enabled them to cope with the scale of their task, and it allowed them to take a overview which encompassed the aims of the educational programme, the needs of the student, the skills and strengths of the people available, and the influences of, and opportunities for learning within, the clinical setting.

For any educational manager role to be effective in the education of the 'trainee' or student, there should be various components. For example, this person needs: to ensure that other practitioners within the organization generally and deliberately act as models or examples for the learner; to have the ability to draw on resources, especially other people, in the provision of educational opportunities for the learner; and above all to possess a clear conception of what is required to develop the learning environment. In these respects, the manager needs sufficient status, power, authority and the requisite skills both organizationally and in terms of being able to theorize.

The concept of the lecturer practitioner seems to be especially valuable when viewed in these terms. Indeed, this has analogies with other professional education roles; for example within teaching and medical education (cf. with the role of the professional tutor in the Oxford Internship Scheme; McIntyre, 1990). Lecturer practitioners can be educational managers of practice *par excellence* in that they are skilled educators and practitioners, with the required credibility and expertise in both settings – the educational institution and the clinical area. None the less, for this to be a viable and effective role it is important for the lecturer practitioner to have power within the clinical setting, but this is power of a particular kind. For example, it would include the ability and authority to select, prepare and support those people with whom the students work most closely (the mentors) as well as the right to remove the student from a clinical area deemed unfit as a learning environment. Without this power, the lecturer practitioner is little more than a lecturer with some clinical knowledge, or a clinical teacher with clinical credibility but no authority. In addition, such a role would allow the lecturer practitioner to take the kind of conceptual overview which is crucially necessary if they are going to achieve a dialectic of theory and practice.

It is argued that it would be feasible for the lecturer practitioner to act in this capacity without necessarily being the manager of practice as well. Rather, the emphasis is on being able to command the resources necessary for effective education. For this to happen, it may be necessary for the lecturer practitioner to be an accepted member of the managerial team.

Dividing the tasks appropriately

Underpinning the concept of lecturer practitioner as being developed here lies the notion of the most appropriate division of labour or, to put it another way, the idea that everyone should be doing what they are best placed to do, but in an integrated way. It was evident that three separate types of planned and actual role in relation to student learning were evident – those of lecturer, mentor and lecturer practitioner – though the precise nature of the differences was not clear in the plans nor, from the in-depth study, were the distinctions between the lecturer and lecturer practitioner roles.

This meant that the original concept from the early documentation of a dichotomy (lecturers and lecturer practitioners) was replaced with a trichotomy or triumvirate – lecturers, lecturer practitioners and mentors. However, viewed in terms of the best division of tasks, this can be very appropriate. Thus, mentors can demonstrate the importance of contextualized practice, work on a day-to-day basis with students and provide the on-going clinical teaching. Lecturers, with their responsibility for theory modules, can articulate theoretical knowledge which provides an up-to-date and research-based framework for students to understand the practice of nursing. And lecturer practitioners, with their educational expertise and their knowledge of the particular context, are in a good position to straddle the two worlds of academia and practice, relating to mentors on the one hand and drawing on theoretical knowledge as it applies to a specialised aspect of nursing on the other, whilst ensuring the positive learning environment in the practice setting.

As such, lecturer practitioners are ideally placed to transform the theory in order for it to interact with practice in a particular context and, as educational managers of practice, they assume a responsibility for the facilitation of the integration between the contributions and actions of the other two partners, though effective integration does depend on the negotiation of a shared agenda between the three. This same argument can be applied to the role of the lecturer practitioner as an assessor of practice. Clearly, in order to assess effectively, there is a need to be in touch with both the practice context and the objectives of the course.

As discussed in the literature review, traditionally clinical education was deemed to be the province of the ward sister or trained nurse allocated to the learner. The early plans for lecturer practitioners suggested that lecturer practitioners would replace sisters in areas used for the 'training' of nurses, and in effect would be the clinical educator. However, in terms of the educational and assessor aspects, (as opposed to their clinical or managerial functions) the reality was that lecturer practitioners provided an extra role, rather than the envisaged replacement role.

This appears to be consistent with UKCC's proposals for the 'Future of Professional Practice' (UKCC, 1994) whereby the concepts of 'advanced nursing practice' and 'specialist nurse practitioners' are being promoted. Advanced nursing practice is envisaged as being concerned with

> adjusting the boundaries for the development of future practice, pioneering and developing new roles responsive to changing needs to enrich professional practice as a whole. (UKCC, 1994, p.8)

Within this 'important sphere' of advanced nursing practice, it is envisaged that there will be specialist practitioners who

> will demonstrate higher levels of clinical decision making and will be able to monitor and improve standards of care through supervision of practice, clinical nursing audit, developing and leading practice, contributing to research, teaching and supporting professional colleagues. (UKCC, 1994, p. 7)

It is unclear from these proposals whether these advanced practitioners will be additional roles, or will, for example, lead to a new 'sister' role. Nevertheless, a lecturer practitioner role – albeit with the modifications and provisos discussed at length in this chapter – could fit well with such proposals.

Resources and conditions

This idea of the lecturer practitioner being additional rather than an alternative to other roles may well have resource implications – depending on such issues as skill mix. Further, the difficulties experienced by the lecturer practitioners in making the job workable imply the necessity for certain conditions (which the survey showed were not always prevalent) and resources: for example, key leadership roles in the planning and evaluation of the course; power within the practice domain to draw on resources required in the education of students), and the time to achieve this effectively. Indeed, the way in which some of the lecturer practitioner roles were organized, especially in terms of the multitude of responsibilities, the expectations, the type and extent of clinical input, and the power to negotiate the role in this respect, and the competing pressures and demands, militated against their effectiveness as practice-based educators and practitioners. It seems to have been a recipe for failure in some instances.

Thus, it is suggested that whilst the principle of practice-based, practice-oriented professional education is sound, attention needs to be paid to the necessary conditions required. Further, it is argued that the present organization of some lecturer practitioner roles does not lend itself well to a viable job, and these are clearly concerns that others taking on the lecturer practitioner concept will need to address.

In conclusion, it can be argued that the concept of lecturer practitioner – as exemplified in this context – has inherent strengths and weaknesses. On the one hand, the idea of a lecturer practitioner as educational manager of practice is powerful, though the conditions necessary for this role would need to be in place. On the other hand, the suggestion that lecturer practitioners should bridge a theory– practice gap is flawed, since this is based on a misconception of 'the theory–practice problem': the proper concerns are multi-dimensional (e.g. conceptual, operational and philosophical amongst others) rather than uni-dimensional.

Further, the aim should not be for integration in the sense of attempting to achieve a seamlessness between theory and practice, but for holding theory and practice in creative tension. If this alternative conception is accepted, then lecturer practitioners have some definite advantages; for example, their location in both the practice and education arenas which facilitates an understanding of both practice and theory concerns; the acceptance by educators and practitioners of the legitimacy of the lecturer practitioners' knowledge and expertise within both practice and education settings; their seniority – the formal and informal authority commanded; and the analytical skills possessed. In the middle ground, the notion of three different but complementary roles is persuasive, and a clear case for the three can be made.

The concept of the lecturer practitioner, as has been understood, has been developed to a very large degree by lecturer practitioners who have been studied working within a particular scheme. Therefore, importantly, the concept has been shaped by them in order to be viable in that context, and this may have resulted in it having certain weaknesses as well as strengths. If this conception of the lecturer practitioner role were to be abstracted and an attempt made to apply it within another setting, new questions would arise. In order to make generalizations beyond this scheme, it is necessary to be aware that the peculiarities and idiosyncrasies of another context will influence the viability and significance of the concept. However, many of the issues that these lecturer practitioner roles have addressed will be the same elsewhere, especially as nurse education and nursing across the country is experiencing the same pressures of major change and upheaval.

Reviewing the role

The collection of data for the research that forms the basis for this text was completed in 1994. The currency of the findings could therefore be challenged. However, a review of the role undertaken in 1996 showed that many of the same issues were still pertinent, albeit to a different extent. The review drew on a variety of sources of information, including discussions and separate reviews undertaken by various of the Trusts, interviews and workshops with LPs, and a series of interviews with Chief Executives and Directors of Nursing. In an unpublished report, Hemphill *et al.* (1996) indicated seven key aspects requiring attention: authority and clinical management responsibility; employment arrangements; the expectations of the Trusts and the University; role outcomes and integration; research and scholarly activity; stress; and career structure.

The clinical management role of LPs

In part, the suggestions in the review reinforced the findings of both the survey and in-depth study in that they showed there to be pros and cons to the different models and managerial arrangements for the lecturer practitioner role. For example, the development of an effective collegiate role was felt to be dependent upon the lecturer practitioner and senior nurse colleagues sharing the same philosophy and having a good working relationship, and the presence of sufficient power to influence decision-making. Given this, the positive aspects of the role were the objectivity (through not being seen as the 'boss'), the 'authority' gained through respect and credibility rather than through line management, and the fact of not having to manage the budget and meet contracts, with their consequent time and financial limitations.

However, in the review, Chief Executives and Directors of Nursing were shown not to favour the combined Unit Manager and LP role in highly acute areas with a fast throughput and in large Units, unless the lecturer practitioner had very good support. It was deemed, nevertheless, to be more workable in smaller, longer stay, Units and to offer the advantage of the authority to develop the Unit and improve the learning environment. In addition, the lecturer practitioner as an advanced practitioner and clinical nurse specialist was promoted more strongly than was found in the research.

Employment arrangements

Though concerns about employment arrangements were not very prevalent in the research findings, they were frequently discussed in the LP forum and other public domains. In the review, they surfaced more overtly. The root of the problem was attributed to the existence of two employers – the Trust and the University. This caused confusion and perceived inequities for some lecturer practitioners, especially in terms of pay and grading, and appointment and appraisal (which are not always clearly the responsibility of either institution). In addition, some lecturer practitioners felt they did not 'belong' to either institution.

Expectations

The related issue of feeling torn between service and education demands was evident in the research and mentioned again in the review. In the latter it was a not infrequent comment by Directors of Nursing that the lecturer practitioners' education role took priority. Conversely, some lecturer practitioners were unhappy about the opposite – that clinical practice demands could make for difficulties in fulfilling their education commitments.

Role outcomes and integration

The opportunity was taken in the review to clarify the education and practice aspects of the role upon which there was agreement. Thus, the suggestion was made that lecturer practitioners had an impact on practice by: leading innovations in practice and Trust-wide projects; challenging practice and improving standards; stimulating nurses to review their practice; and spreading the ethos that education is part of everyone's job.

In addition, lecturer practitioners were considered to integrate theory and practice by a variety of means, including: educating whilst practising (being a recognized education resource); helping staff and students make connections between theory and practice; modelling expertise when with clients and families; using reflection as a tool for learning; thinking laterally; and encouraging professional awareness.

In terms of integrating all aspects of the role, however, there was a general view that it was impossible to be an expert in all four dimensions (practice, education, management and research) or to do them all at once. This was expressed by managers ('the role is too enormous for one person') and reinforced by LPs' own expressed feelings of discomfort and guilt at not doing everything. In reality, lecturer practitioners focused on one or two aspects at any one time, just as they had done in the period of the research. The issue remained, though, of the lack of understanding of this necessity, leading at times to unrealistic expectations.

Research and scholarly activity

The ways of fostering research identified by the review were identical to those found in the in-depth study and survey – for example, encouraging research-based practice; undertaking research as part of a course; and supporting others doing research. Nevertheless, the review suggested that the model of research that lecturer practitioners were commonly engaged in was that of internal evaluation, as described by Lathlean (1995b). Yet whilst lecturer practitioners considered this to be useful in terms of developing practice and the learning environment, it appeared to be an activity that was neither recognized nor valued by the Trust and the University.

Stress

The research had highlighted many stressors in the role, and these were deemed still to be prevalent, notably: being pulled in different directions; high workload and hours; appraisal mechanisms; pressures of change; lack of resources and support; inadequate role orientation. Nevertheless, it was recognized that improvements in some factors (e.g. better orientation and support) could lead to a greater ability to cope with other aspects, such as high workload demands, thereby reducing stress.

Career structure

The final concern was that of a lack of career structure. Whilst the LP role was seen as valuable in that it allowed experienced clinical nurses to progress whilst retaining their expertise, the question of 'what next' for the LPs themselves was raised. Though not identified by the research or the review, it is known that several lecturer practitioners have left the role to take on even more challenging and demanding roles for the individuals, such as full-time research roles, and management positions where the ability to have a direct impact on practice has been built into the job.

The review concludes by arguing that there is a strong commitment to maintaining the original concept of integrating the education and practice remit within one job, and in developing the lecturer practitioner role to strengthen both this aspect and that of the role of lecturer practitioner as facilitator of learning through reflection.

The lecturer practitioner role in other settings

Whilst the lecturer practitioner role was being implemented in this setting – and since this time – the role has spread in popularity throughout the country. Although lecturer practitioner type posts are becoming increasingly more common in academic and Trust settings, much of the comment upon the roles is anecdotal and not evidence-based. There appear to be no published evaluation research studies of the role as such, but two pieces of work are of particular interest. The first is described as a one-year feasibility study to look at the implementation aspects of the lecturer practitioner role (in nursing), it is set within the West Midlands Region, and involves interviews with 29 people, six of whom purport to be occupying a lecturer practitioner role (Jones, 1994). The second is a six-month investigation to compile a database of the distribution and scope of lecture practitioner roles in Trent Region, and focuses on 30 (of the 36) LPs in post in that region (Fairbrother and Ford, 1996).

There are considerable similarities between the findings of these two reports and between the reports and the research. For example, on the positive side, in line with the research, both studies argue that the lecturer practitioner role at a minimum has key responsibilities spanning the education and practice arenas and is thought effective for 'enhancing and forging a closer relationship between service and education' (Fairbrother and Ford, 1996). Similarly, they both make a plea for an extension and expansion of the lecturer practitioner role. In terms of improvements required, the need for role clarity is implied or stated, with Jones (1994) recommending that managers need to work through the purpose of a role when new posts are being created, and Fairbrother and Ford (1996) maintaining that the success of lecturer practitioners 'hinges upon a clear understanding of those parties involved in the post'.

In addition, both refer to the need for support mechanisms within the organization for these innovative post, with Jones (1994) urging the establishment of a national support system. Similarly, the importance of preparation for the role and the issue of career development within and beyond the lecturer practitioner post was mentioned by the two studies. Both reports also urge that, despite the shared philosophy behind the different lecturer practitioner posts, they should be viewed as context-specific and developed in line with the particular characteristics and needs of the setting within which they are located. This was a key finding of the research as well.

Where the reports differ from each other is in Jones' emphasis on the prerequisite criteria for lecturer practitioners, including minimum qualifications and experience – a diploma in nursing, an approved educational qualification and ward management experience; the existence of certain (somewhat self-evident) personal characteristics such as good communication and inter-personal skills, assertiveness, empathy and flexibility; and the absence of other traits, such as lethargy, lack of competence and credibility, and being a follower, not a leader. And Fairbrother and Ford, perhaps as a result of the increasing pre-occupations of Trusts and educational institutions with value for money and evidence of outcomes, include in their study the need of purchasers to be persuaded of the value of a lecturer practitioner post and the requirement of lecturer practitioners therefore 'to be sufficiently skilled in order to demonstrate value for money within these different cultures' (Fairbrother and Ford, 1996 p. 42). Their call also for evaluative studies reflects the previously mentioned theme of the need for greater role clarity in order to establish criteria against which performance can be measured.

The future

This text has concentrated on the implementation and development of the lecturer practitioner role and the messages are clear – that it is a role with considerable merit and one that warrants expansion. Nevertheless, it is only one approach to the problem, albeit that, as stressed throughout, there are many different variants – there is in reality no one lecturer practitioner role. It must be viewed in the context of the increasing emphasis on the role of the nurse teacher in practice, as well as within the climate of a desire for better collaboration between the practice of nursing and the education of novices and professional development of nurses. In addition, there are considerations raised by the emphasis on the purchaser and provider split and with the changed managerial arrangements and service and education expectations.

In the setting for the research, the choice was to go down the road of embedding lecturer practitioners in large numbers within the nursing management structure as well as the new education structure. This required major changes both in the way that education was delivered and in clinical roles. Elsewhere, lecturer practitioners are being introduced within existing structures and on a post-by-post basis. Whilst this can be problematic it also offers the possibility for exploring other innovative solutions such as support roles for lecturer practitioners (sometimes known as link teachers, associate lecturers or even super mentors) as well as nurse teachers with enhanced practice roles. In addition, the specific contextual needs can be thoroughly explored.

Clearly it is important to learn from the experience of others so as not to re-invent the wheel, nor to fall into the same traps as many past attempts at addressing the key issues of theory and practice in nursing have done. It is hoped that through this sortie into the world of lecturer practitioners, the insights gained will be of interest and value – not just to those in the role and those considering them, but also to anyone who is concerned about improving professional practice and education and their interconnections.

References

Aamodt, A. M. (1991) Ethnography and epistemology: generating nursing knowledge. In Morse, J. M. (Ed) *Qualitative Nursing Research: A Contemporary Dialogue*, Sage Publications, Newbury Park, CA

Agar M. H. (1980) *The Professional Stranger: An Informal Introduction to Ethnography*, Academic Press Inc, Orlando, FL

Alexander, M. F. (1980) Nurse Education: An Experiment in Integration of Theory and Practice in Nursing. Unpublished PhD Thesis, University of Edinburgh

Alexander, M. F. (1983) *Learning to Nurse: Integrating Theory and Practice*, Churchill Livingstone, Edinburgh

Atkinson, P. and Hammersley, M. (1994) Ethnography and participant observation. In Denzin, N. K. and Lincoln, Y. S. (Eds) *Handbook of Qualitative Research*, Sage Publications, Newbury Park, CA

Benner, P. (1984) *From Novice to Expert: Excellence and Power in Clinical Nursing Practice*, Addison-Wesley, Menlo Park, CA

Bryman, A. (1988) *Quantity and Quality in Social Research*, Unwin Hyman, London

Bulmer, M. (1979) Concepts in the analysis of qualitative data. Sociological Review, Vol. 27, No. 3, pp. 651–77

Cahill, M. (1993) *Effective Nursing – an Exploration by Experienced Nurses*, Ashdale Press, Oxford

Champion, R. (1988) Competent Nurse? Reflective Practitioner? Unpublished paper, International Conference on Nursing Education, Cardiff

Champion, R. (1989) Nursing Education in the 1990s. Unpublished paper, National Nursing Conference, Ulster

Denzin, N. K. (1978) *The Research Act: A Theoretical Introduction to Sociological Methods*, Second Edition, McGraw-Hill, New York

Department of Health and Social Security (1972) *Report of the Committee on Nursing* (Chairman: Briggs), HMSO, London

Fairbrother, P. and Ford, S. (1996) *Mapping the Territory – Lecturer Practitioners in Trent. Report to the NHS Executive Trent*, University of Sheffield, School of Nursing and Midwifery, Sheffield

George, P. (1987) The Nurse as a Reflective Practitioner. Unpublished Paper, Department of Social Studies, Oxford Polytechnic

Glaser, B. and Strauss, A. L. (1967) *The Discovery of Grounded Theory: Strategies for Qualitative Research*, Aldine, Chicago

Goetz, J. P. and LeCompte, M. D. (1984) *Ethnography and Qualitative Design in Educational Research*, Academic Press, Orlando, FL

Gold, R. L. (1958) Roles in sociological fieldwork. *Social Forces*, Vol. 36, pp. 217–23

Gott, M. (1984) *Learning Nursing*, Royal College of Nursing, London

Guba, E. G. and Lincoln, Y. S. (1982) Epistemological and methodological bases of naturalistic enquiry. *Educational Communication and Technology Journal*, Vol. 30, No. 4, pp. 232–55

Gumpertz, J. (1981) Conversational inference and classroom learning. In Green, J. L. and Wallat, C. (Eds) *Ethnography and Language in Educational Settings*, Ablex, Norwood, NY

Hammersley, M. and Atkinson, P. (1983) *Ethnography. Principles in Practice*, Tavistock Publications, London

Hemphill, A., Muir, J. and Whitehead, L. (1996) Review of the Lecturer Practitioner Role. Unpublished report on behalf of the Lecturer Practitioner Forum. Oxford Brookes University, School of Health Care Studies, Oxford

Jacka, K. and Lewin, D. (1987) *The Clinical Learning of Student Nurses*, Nursing Education Research Unit, King's College, University of London

Jones, H. M. (1994) Implementation Aspects of the Lecturer-Practitioner Role. A Report for the West Midlands Regional Health Authority. Unpublished Report

Judge, H. (1980) Teaching and professionalisation: an essay in ambiguity. In Hoyle, E. and Megarry, J. (Eds) *World Yearbook of Education 1980: Professional Development*, Kogan Page, London

Kuhn, T. S. (1962) *The Structure of Scientific Revolutions*, Second Edition, University of Chicago Press, Chicago

Lathlean, J. (1994a) Choosing an appropriate methodology. In Buckeldee, J. and McMahon, R. *The Research Experience in Nursing*, Chapman and Hall, London

Lathlean, J. (1994b) Historical and empirical approaches. In Lathlean, J. and Vaughan, B. (Eds) *Unifying Nursing Practice and Theory*, Butterworth Heinemann, Oxford

Lathlean, J. (1995a) *The Implementation and Development of Lecturer Practitioners in Nursing* (DPhil Thesis), Ashdale Press, Oxford

Lathlean, J. (1995b) *Interface Between Research and Practice: Some Working Models. An Executive Summary*, Kings Fund, London

Lathlean, J. and Farnish, S. (1984) *The Ward Sister Training Project*, Nursing Education Research Unit, Chelsea College, University of London

Lathlean, J., Smith, G. and Bradley, S. (1986) *Post-Registration Development Schemes Evaluation*, NERU Report No. 4, King's College, University of London

LeCompte, M. D. and Goetz, J. P. (1982) Problems of reliability and validity in ethnographic research. *Review of Educational Research*, Vol. 52, No. 1, pp. 31–60

Lofland, J. (1971) *Analyzing Social Settings: A Guide to Qualitative Observation and Analysis*, Wadsworth Publishing Company, Belmont, CA

Lofland, J. and Lofland, L. H. (1984) *Analyzing Social Settings: A Guide to Qualitative Observation and Analysis*, Second Edition, Wadsworth Publishing Company, Belmont, CA

Lutz, F. W. (1981) Ethnography – the holistic approach to understanding schooling. In Green, J. L and Wallat, C. (Eds) *Ethnography and Language in Educational Settings*, Ablex, Norwood, NY

MacLeod, M. (1990) Experience in Everyday Nursing Practice. A Study of 'Experienced' Ward Sisters. Unpublished PhD Thesis, University of Edinburgh

Martin, L. (1989) *Clinical Education in Perspective*, Royal College of Nursing, London

McCaugherty, D. (1991a) The use of a teaching model to promote reflection and the experiential integration of theory and practice in first-year student nurses: an action research study. *Journal of Advanced Nursing*, Vol. 16, pp. 534–43

McCaugherty, D. (1991b) The theory practice gap in nurse education: its causes and possible solutions. Findings from an action research study. *Journal of Advanced Nursing*, Vol. 16, pp. 1055–61

McIntyre, D. (1990) Ideas and principles guiding the internship scheme. In Benton, P. (Ed) *The Oxford Internship Scheme: Integration and Partnership in Initial Teacher Education*, Calouste Gulbenkian Foundation, London

Melia, K. M. (1981) Student Nurses' Accounts of their Work and Training: A Qualitative Analysis. Unpublished PhD Thesis, University of Edinburgh

Melia, K. M. (1982) 'Tell it as it is' – qualitative methodology and nursing research: understanding the student nurse's world. *Journal of Advanced Nursing*, Vol. 7, pp. 327–35

Melia, K. M. (1987) *Learning and Working: The Occupational Socialization of Nurses*, Tavistock Publications, London

Mitchell, J. C. (1983) Case and situation analysis. *The Sociological Review*, Vol. 31, No. 2, pp. 187-211

Patton, M. Q. (1990) *Qualitative Evaluation and Research Methods*, Second Edition, Sage Publications, Newbury Park, CA

Pelto, P. J. and Pelto, G. H. (1978) *Anthropological Research: The Structure of Inquiry*, Second Edition, Cambridge University Press, Cambridge

Rafferty, A. M., Alcock, N. and Lathlean, J. (1996) The theory/practice 'gap'; taking issue with the issue. *Journal of Advanced Nursing*, 23, 685–91

Rapoport, R. and Rapoport, R. N. (1976) *Dual Career Families Re-examined*, Martin Robertson, London

Reid, N. G. (1983) A Multivariate Statistical Investigation of the Factors Affecting Nurse Training in the Clinical Area. Unpublished PhD Thesis, New University of Ulster

Reid, N. G. (1985) *Wards in Chancery? Nurse Training in the Clinical Area*, Royal College of Nursing, London

Robertson, C. M. (1987) *A Very Special Form of Teaching*, Royal College of Nursing, London

Royal College of Nursing (1985) *The Education of Nurses: A New Dispensation. Commission on Nursing Education* (Chairman: Judge), Royal College of Nursing, London

Royal Commission on the National Health Service (1979) *Royal Commission on the National Health Service* (Merrison Report), HMSO (Cmnd 7615), London

Schön, D. (1983) *The Reflective Practitioner: How Professionals Think in Action*, Temple Smith, London

Schön, D. (1987) *Educating the Reflective Practitioner: Towards a New Design for Teaching and Learning in the Professions*, Jossey-Bass Publishers, San Francisco, CA

Schutz, A. (1964) The stranger: an essay in social psychology. In Schutz, A. (Ed) Collected Papers, Vol. II, Martinus Nijhoff, The Hague

Schutz, A. (1972) *The Phenomenology of the Social World*, Heinemann Educational Books, London

Silverman, D. (1985) *Qualitative Methodology and Sociology*, Gower, Aldershot

Spradley, J. P. (1979) *The Ethnographic Interview*, Rinehart & Winston, New York

Spradley, J. P. (1980) *Participant Observation*, Rinehart & Winston, New York

Strauss, A. and Corbin, J. (1990) *Basics of Qualitative Research. Grounded Theory Procedures and Techniques*, Sage Publications, London

United Kingdom Central Council For Nursing, Midwifery and Health Visiting (1986) *Project 2000: A New Preparation for Practice*, UKCC, London

United Kingdom Central Council For Nursing, Midwifery and Health Visiting (1994) *The Future of Professional Practice – the Council's Standards for Education and Practice Following Registration*. Position Statement on Policy and Implementation, March 1994, UKCC, London

Vaughan, B. (1987) Bridging the gap – teaching roles in nurse education. *Senior Nurse*, Vol. 6, No. 5, pp. 30–1

Vaughan, B. (1988) Teaching Roles in Nurse Education. Unpublished paper. International Conference on Nursing Education, Cardiff

Vaughan, B. (1989) Two roles – one job. *Nursing Times*, Vol. 85, No. 11, p. 52

Vaughan, B. (1990) Knowing that and knowing how: the role of the lecturer practitioner. In Kershaw, B. and Salvage, J. (Eds) *Models for Nursing 2*, Scutari Press, London

Walker, R. (1981) On the uses of fiction in educational research. In Smetherham, D. (Ed) *Practising Evaluation*, Nafferton, Driffield

Wright, S. G. (1981) The Role of the Clinical Teacher in General Nursing. Unpublished MSc Thesis, University of Manchester.

Index